WILLIAM D. ESTEB

CHIROPRACTIC

PATIENTOLOGY

◀◀◀◀ ▶▶▶▶

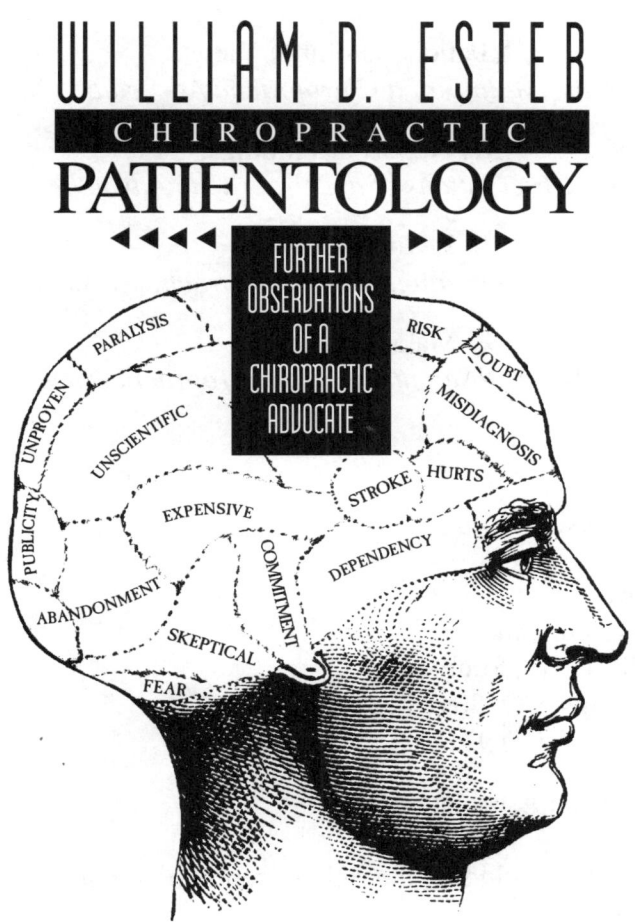

FURTHER
OBSERVATIONS
OF A
CHIROPRACTIC
ADVOCATE

Also by William D. Esteb

A Patient's Point of View,
Observations of a Chiropractic Advocate

My Report of Findings,
More Observations of a Chiropractic Advocate

Beyond Results,
Still More Observations of a Chiropractic Advocate

Making Change,
Even Still More Observations of a Chiropractic Advocate

Published by
Orion Associates, Inc.

Distributed by
Back Talk Systems, Inc.
2845 Ore Mill Drive, Suite 4
Colorado Springs, CO 80904-3161
(719) 633-1105 (800) 937-3113

Cover designed by Buffalo Brothers, Inc.
Manufactured in the United States of America

Esteb, William D., 1952 -

Chiropractic Patientology
Further Observations of a Chiropractic Advocate
ISBN 0-9631711-4-3

For the chiropractic pioneers who went to jail for chiropractic.

TABLE OF CONTENTS

FOREWORD

Bill Esteb has written a very timely and insightful book which will assist many chiropractors in navigating the rough seas that lay ahead in the health care marketplace. A prolific writer and thinker, Bill presents to his readers, in this, his fifth book, a valuable guide to keeping in tune and on track, maintaining a positive vision and attitude, despite the confusion and turmoil which characterizes the sweeping changes we all face in the competitive, increasingly managed-care dominated, marketplace.

With a wry wit, he prods his readers to the edge of their comfort zone, asking them to confront the reality that the once secure and insurance-financed abundance of the 1980s is history. He illustrates, with many amusing examples, why yesterday's solutions no longer answer the needs of today's crises and offers practical, yet inspiring, suggestions to help as we move toward the threshold of the next century.

In the 1980s, chiropractors were lulled into a false sense of security by the ready reimbursement provided by insurance equality and personal injury coverage. Reimbursement for our services caused the costs, of what became largely symptomatic care, to soar. Today, unfortunately, both insurance and personal injury coverage seem to be evaporating before our eyes, so patient education becomes an even more essential cornerstone of the successful practice.

In order to thrive in an otherwise uncertain future, we must regain and communicate our enthusiasm and excitement for the principles and benefits of chiropractic. This is made even easier today with the profusion of evidence in the current scientific literature documenting the effectiveness, safety, and enormously high patient satisfaction with chiropractic care. If communicated clearly, and explained with metaphors patients understand, it is easy for them to appreciate the value of our approach to health which emphasizes optimal function and well-being. Through his experience with patient focus groups, Esteb offers us crucial insights into patients' perspectives on chiropractic and provides us with many methods by which to enhance their understanding, compliance, and increased referrals by patients taught to communicate the benefits of chiropractic.

This very readable book offers us, in an original and entertaining format, solutions to current challenges, tools for confronting our personal limitations which will serve us well, long into the future.

Malik Slosberg, D.C., M.S.
Pleasanton, California

INTRODUCTION

D. D. Palmer said, "There are only two classes in the world, Doctors and Patients". Is it not wise to understand just how patients think, how they view us, how they interpret our explanations?

William Esteb speaks as a knowledgeable chiropractic advocate. He began, of course as a patient, seeing the need for chiropractors to increase their skills in communication with patients. He began his successful program of educating chiropractors on just how to clearly bring forth the principles of our separate and distinct health care paradigm.

You see, this is chiropractic's age of responsibility. Our juvenile and adolescent years are behind us. Directly proportionate to our ability to communicate our wellness model, will be the degree of prosperity and acceptance we will achieve in the twenty-first century. The public yearns for our model of health care. We have the design they seek—but we must articulate our chiropractic principles with clarity. And this has been particularly difficult for us.

This is where Bill Esteb comes in. He explains the perceived risks people see in coming under chiropractic care. Perceived value must overshadow perceived risks if the person is to become a chiropractic patient. He lucidly explains the many aspects of the patients understanding and needs. Chapter after chapter he attacks areas of concern. He teaches us to cast off bad habits and don a new coat of consciousness, not only in respect to doctor patient relationships, but our own perception of the worthiness and value of chiropractic.

You will find no gimmicks herein. He seeks to educate us in

3

communicative skills, how to develop an informed and participatory staff, and his words are delivered with authority, honesty, and integrity.

I need say no more. I find Bill Esteb's writings thought provoking and above all useful and worthwhile. He shares my dream of bringing this profession to the pinnacle of achievement it deserves. He speaks of the role we play in health—the doctor, the patient, and the doctor's staff.

I will close in the words of B. J. Palmer, who would say as you begin this book, "enter to learn how."

"Enuf" said,

Fred H. Barge, D.C., Ph.C.
(Hon)FICA,FPAC,SCS
La Crosse, Wisconsin

SPECIAL THANKS

As with previous volumes, the ideas presented here are heavily influenced by the hundreds of doctors and staff members I've met at seminars and talked with over the telephone. If my words touch a responsive chord in you, it is due to the countless doctors who have openly shared their fears and frustrations.

This is the year I discovered the internet and I thank Paul Cronshaw, D.C. for his urging to do so. It is always difficult to embrace something new and I appreciate his coaxing and "cyberspace savvy."

I thank everyone at Back Talk Systems, Inc., especially my partner Robert Jackson, D.C. for being such a great confidant and friend. You helped polish these ideas by the inspirational example you set in your life and in your practice.

Thanks to my editors, Dusty Sorrentino and Andrea Ramsauer, the grammar is clearer than it would have been. Perhaps more important, their encouragement provided the impetus to trust myself during the exploration of some of the more sensitive areas contained herein.

Finally, thanks to Marilyn, Eric, and Marylou who provide a daily reality check and who's love and support make what I do possible in the first place.

William D. Esteb
Colorado Springs, Colorado

DEAR DR. BROWN

I'm sure by now you've realized that I've decided to stop receiving chiropractic care in your office. You probably drew this conclusion from the exceedingly long time that has passed since my last visit, or most certainly by the request to have my X-rays sent elsewhere. Due to the circumstances, I didn't have the opportunity to sit down with you and explain my decision. Since I have such a high regard for you, I want to take this opportunity to explain my actions.

We go back a long way. You were the second chiropractor we had, switching to your office back in 1982 when you had just opened your doors. I know that you and chiropractic care played at least some part in the miracle of Eric's conception and birth, and for that I will be forever thankful. Those were heady days for me and chiropractic! The videos. Disneyworld. The excitement of being part of something big.

Your office naturally grew. Your excellent adjusting skills, passion for chiropractic, and sincere interest in each patient made your practice a welcome oasis for me, my family, and countless other patients. Yet, as more patients discovered chiropractic through you, office visits became interminably long. Even with your three adjusting rooms, when the waiting time became 45 minutes or more, I opted to seek chiropractic care elsewhere. While I was uncomfortable "abandoning" you, I couldn't afford to pay for my care twice, first for your wonderful adjustments, and second, in the form of lost time. I think you admitted that office procedures and practice capacity had become a challenge, and that you had sought advice for improvements. I noticed those improvements upon returning to your office these last several years. However, my most recent departure from your office has nothing to do with reception room waiting time.

One of the many challenges of any small business person is hiring staff, setting fees, and establishing business hours. These are decisions that are difficult to make and are rarely determined the first time around. While I've always felt your fee structure was extremely fair, staffing and office hours are more troubling.

Since my schedule rarely affords me the opportunity to set appointment times in advance, I attempt to identify the slowest times of the day and week and show up then. Clearly, your staff doesn't like walk-ins! Did I mess up her perfectly choreographed appointment book? Was I perceived as disrespectful by not making appointments, even though regardless of appointments, patients are seen on a first come, first served basis?

I know Linda brings some valuable skills to your office. I'm sure her organizational skills and analytical perspective help bring some order to the chaos of running a busy practice like yours. Only problem is, your front desk person is not a people person! Which is one of the most important skills someone who makes the most lasting first and last impression of your office must have.

But, I can look beyond the obvious personality difference I have with her. What pushed me over the edge was showing up for care and finding you gone. Seminar, vacation, special circumstances at home; there was always an excuse. I don't begrudge your desire to have a life, however, I got tired of making the effort to get to your office, and finding *you* hadn't taken the effort to get to your office.

It has certainly occurred to me that I may be a patient you're not interested in having in your practice. Changing office hours and taking unscheduled month-long vacations might just be a low-confrontational way of shaking patients like me who only show up once or twice a month, paying your affordable cash fee for wellness care. Perhaps wellness/maintenance patients are too boring? Or are not profitable enough?

Whether it was a conscious decision on your part, or just a series of unfortunate circumstances, I wanted you to know that I have the highest regard for your clinical skills and that I believe that I have received excellent care from you. It's just that I need a chiropractor with office hours more predictable than my own.

Warmest regards,

William D. Esteb

THE PERFECT STAFF

Probably the most telling aspects of a doctor's relationship with patients is the relationship between the doctor and his or her staff. Staff relationships reveal a lot about the doctor's communication skills, management savvy, and personality defects. Doctors who are most successful in growing long-term relationships with patients, seem adroit in their relationships with staff members. Yet, there is a fundamental difference: patients pay the doctor, but the doctor pays the staff. So staff members are more likely than patients to put up with a doctor's shortcomings. Conversely, because staff members know that it is impolite to bite the hand that feeds them, they are reluctant to criticize or tell the emperor that he's not wearing any clothes. Dysfunctional doctor/staff relationships continue to blunt the impact of many chiropractic offices.

In Hal Rosenbluth's book, *The Customer Comes Second*, this issue is addressed in the context of one of the world's largest travel agencies. Mr. Rosenbluth's perspective that the needs of the staff come *before* the needs of the customer (patient), flies in the face of conventional wisdom. It is tempting to look past the staff and focus entirely on the patient, the patient's spine, the patient's form of payment, and the patient's likes and dislikes. And while it's important in this age of "consumerism" to be responsive to the needs of patients, bypassing the staff can sabotage even the best laid plans for your patients.

Yet, because effective staff hiring, training, and management are not taught in chiropractic college, this void is filled by entrepreneurial forces who often teach a form of hierarchal staff management based on fear, intimidation, and isolation. A management style that is even more ineffective and out of touch than it was in the early 1950s when it captured the imagination of General Motors, IBM, and other corporate behemoths.

Based on the conversations I've had with staff members on the telephone, or in seminar situations when the doctor is out of earshot, an interesting profile emerges.

No training. It's astonishing, that with the critical role staff members play in the service to patients, that they are so poorly trained. When I ask staff members on the telephone what adjusting techniques the doctor uses, many who answer the telephone act as if I've suddenly broken into an esoteric dialect of Portuguese! Basic issues like adjusting technique, which chiropractic college the doctor attended (and when), special training, awards, specialities, financial policies, and other fundamentals should be part of every staff person's understanding. Unfortunately, doctors are rarely in a position to observe staff members fumbling these topics, nor is there a ledger entry that records the loss of patient confidence and practice income these gaffs cause. Apparently, staff training, when it does occur, is the result of occasional management seminars or conducted in the heat of battle while the doctor is distracted by the demands of patient care.

Action steps: Reserve a consistent time each week, maybe a Tuesday or Thursday morning, for staff training and rehearsal. Yes, rehearsal. Remember, products are manufactured, and services like chiropractic are performed. An effective rush hour is as much a performance as it is an issue of being a traffic cop. Practice when the office is empty. Role play at the front desk. Call into the office from the second line and pretend you're a new patient calling 10 minutes before closing time. Ask about fees, appointment times, and generally push the limits. Practice with the actual forms, questions, and environment your staff will encounter on a busy Wednesday evening!

Staff in fear. It's still amazing that there are doctors who think the best way to get staff members to perform is by threats, intimidation, and a fear-based management style. This approach may purchase their bodies, but it ignores their minds. So while staff members dutifully show up one minute before starting time and leave within one minute after closing time, their emotional commitment is missing. They do as they are told, but contribute little else. They offer few, if any suggestions for improvement. They are afraid to approach the doctor or, if appropriate, the doctor's spouse with a problem or concern for fear of being reprimanded or scolded. Little problems fester. The staff is quietly plotting their getaway, always looking for another job. Staff turnover is epidemic under these working conditions.

Action steps: The most contemporary, mainstream management style teaches the importance of empowering the people actually doing the work to help shape the nature of their work. I'm not suggesting turning the asylum over to the inmates! Create an environment where staff members feel comfortable continually rethinking their job responsibilities and looking for ways to improve them. Imagine the countless offices still using the same procedures, the same paperwork, the same scripts, and the same policies as they did six years ago before the decay of indemnity insurance and the emergence of managed care! Institute a policy that invites a continual questioning of the status quo. Reward staff members who are good at asking "why?" and who look for ways to enhance, streamline, or discard inefficiencies and needless effort. The only thing to fear from this management posture is that you may find yourself having to defend procedures whose purpose you've neglected to explain, or discard policies that give you a false sense of security. Get real!

Staff excluded from clinical concerns. Without some knowledge and appreciation for your clinical approaches, not only do you exclude your staff from the joys and fulfillment you experience, but you've tricked them into a boring, dead end job. How long do you think you'd last where the pinnacle of achievement is keeping patient files in alphabetical order, and supervising an appointment book in which the objective is to get patients to show up in an order previously scheduled?

Action steps: Involve your staff in the clinical picture of each new patient. Explain how you approach each case. Reveal the concerns you have. Share your frustrations. Bring your staff into the "inner circle." Sure, they may never fully appreciate the mind-numbing training and classroom work you've had to put up with to get to this place, but try.

Certainly there are issues of patient confidentiality here, but if your staff is too immature to understand and respect these dynamics, you may have the wrong staff. No wonder so many doctors feel isolated in their practices—they haven't groomed any teammates!

Staff given the dirty work. The mark of good leadership is never to assign a task to a subordinate that you wouldn't be willing to do yourself. Yet, all too often, staff members are asked to lie ("He's with patients right now...") or to badger patients to return for care they don't understand or want ("Yeah, the doctor found something on your X-rays he wants to talk to you about...") or perform personal errands that would make even an indentured servant feel uncomfortable. Interestingly, these tasks are rarely discussed during the interview process before staff members are hired.

Action steps: Create some clear job descriptions at your next staff meeting. Outline job functions which are considered daily duties, weekly responsibilities, and occasional tasks. If you're expecting staff members to entertain young children, vacuum the office, and pick up your dry cleaning, let them know in advance. Lots of qualified staff members would be delighted to perform these chores—if your expectations are outlined in advance!

The promise of change. Doctors would be surprised how many staff members dread attending chiropractic seminars. And it's not for the reasons that many doctors think. Many staff members look forward to a little vacation away from their families in a swanky hotel, complete with room service. What they hate is being exposed to lots of great ideas that are never acted upon. What is so disappointing is watching the doctor spend thousands of dollars on a management firm, only to ignore the advice, or giving up after only half-heartedly trying a new procedure for a week or so. After a couple of rah-rah sessions at the Hyatt, in which the promise of change is made, but not acted upon, staff members see what a wimp their doctor is and would rather stay home and do laundry.

Action steps: Make up your mind. Decide. Focus. If your management firm doesn't reflect your values or you're not inclined to act upon the suggestions presented at the next seminar, don't go! If you bring your staff, have every one contribute to a "to do" list when you return, before even the most obvious idea is newly implemented. As a team, decide which ideas have merit and how much time will be needed to confirm their value. Then, implement them with complete and total commitment. Holding back almost assures failure.

Not only do staff members spend more time with patients than the doctor, they make the most enduring, first and last impressions. They set the tone of the office and supervise its environment. They can make patients feel they are either a source of joy, or an irritating, schedule-busting inconvenience. They can spearhead office growth, or they can serve as a governor, regulating practice volume. Besides the ability to adjust patients, there may be no other more important aspect of practice than nurturing a great staff. ■

RISKY BUSINESS

All of us have our own unique level of risk tolerance. At both ends of the "risk" continuum you find the dysfunctional—those willing to gamble the house, the car, and next month's paycheck, or those who hold themselves captive in their own homes, afraid to risk exposure to the uncertainties of walking down the street or being engulfed by a crowd. Between these two extremes is a vast middle ground of people who make decisions and choices using seemingly more temperate guidelines. Some will feel comfortable risking a meal at an exotic Thai restaurant, and others will not. Some will feel comfortable attending a new church, while others will not. Some will risk wearing the latest fashion, while others will not. And some will risk chiropractic care, while others will not.

Chiropractic is risky business.

To a chiropractor with hundreds of successful cases under his or her belt, it may be hard for you to imagine. As a chiropractor knowing and appreciating the simplicity and effectiveness of chiropractic, it's difficult to understand a prospective patient's fears. After thousands, maybe hundreds of thousands of uneventful adjustments, it's virtually impossible to comprehend the fears that an uninitiated patient might have. Meanwhile most chiropractors look on with incredulity, as millions of patients opt to unnecessarily endure pain, go for numbing drugs, or choose surgical intervention instead of chiropractic care. But, it is at this fundamental level of risk tolerance that these seemingly irresponsible patient actions almost make sense.

Patients perceive surgery to be less risky than chiropractic. Patients perceive physical therapy to be less risky than chiropractic. Patients perceive addictive medication to be less risky than chiropractic. Patients perceive doing nothing to be less risky than chiropractic. To the millions of prospective patients who could likely benefit from chiropractic care, they choose not to, because of the perceived risks.

These risks are the enemy of practice growth and professional acceptance. Not the AMA. Not the insurance companies. Not the IMEs. Not the HMOs. Not cost containment. These risks often prevent the investigation of chiropractic in the first place! It is each practitioner's ability to overcome these risks and equip patients to not only defend their chiropractic decision, but to empower them to arrest these fears in others, that affects practice referrals and retention.

Webster defines risk in two ways. Risk, according to one definition is the chance of "incurring harm or danger", and the other is the "possibility of suffering a loss." Some of the more common patient perceived risks from incurring harm or danger are:

- Chiropractic will make my condition worse.
- The chiropractor may overlook something serious.
- The chiropractor will hurt me.
- I'll get a stroke or be paralyzed.

Ironically, these physical risks may not be as influential in the behavior of prospective patients as the "fear of loss." Only when a prospective patient's tolerance for pain is reached, will some patients feel the risks of harm or danger are worth encountering. The notion of risk tolerance may explain why so many patients show up in your office only at the most acute and helpless stages of pain.

Perhaps more powerful than the perceived physical danger of chiropractic, is the psychological or economic risks associated with beginning chiropractic care. Some of the more common patient perceived risks in the "suffering a loss" category include:

- I'll be wasting my time and money (loss of resources)
- My friends will think I'm a fool (loss of acceptance)
- My medical doctor will abandon me (loss of support)
- My insurance/HMO won't reimburse me (loss of finances)
- I'll get addicted to adjustments (loss of control)

Again, for those who have been in the chiropractic subculture for some time, these notions seem so at odds with the truth, that they are easily overlooked or minimized. Those who do, misjudge the potency of these beliefs. Changing these patient-held notions may be more important to the future and growth of your practice than describing subluxations, explaining the associated soft tissue damage, or having a reasonable fee structure.

Based upon this model, you might be correct in assuming that to date, chiropractic has primarily reached those with a relatively high risk tolerance. A common metaphor used to describe this risk index comes from the taming of the "wild west." The first to go out west were those with the highest risk tolerance, the scouts. Followed by the pioneers, and then, only when the risks were minimal, the settlers. For the most part, chiropractic has attracted the scouts and the risk-tolerant pioneers. The settlers haven't shown up yet.

A well educated and informed patient base is one strategy that can help overcome some of these notions. Even with a well-orchestrated public relations program, it may take generations to transform the risky perception of chiropractic that is held by the general population. Until then, make sure you change these notions in the patients who *are* brave enough to venture into your office.

Action steps: Battling the "harm or danger" myth, like overcoming other types of misinformation, requires an aggressive, proactive approach. Go beyond merely posting your college diplomas! Explain the continuing education you receive and what it means to typical patients (state-of-the-art care, safer, more accurate adjustments, etc.). Explain the value of chiropractic X-rays and the patient benefits of taking them (more accurate care, confirmation of other examinations, way to track your progress, etc.). Explain your working relationships with other non-DC health care practitioners; assure patients of your non-dogmatic practice style and that they won't become helpless pawns in an inter-professional battle. Explain the safety issues associated with chiropractic care. Remind patients of the "informed consent" documents one must sign to receive care in a hospital and that chiropractic is so safe, none seem required. Compare the cost of your malpractice insurance premiums with a medical general practitioner down the street. Photocopy pages from the New Zealand government study documenting the "unusually safe" history of chiropractic care.

Action steps: Overcoming the "possibility of incurring a loss" is more challenging. Put your patient's financial concerns at ease by assuming the risk. "I can't guarantee results, but I can guarantee your satisfaction. So if within __ visits you're not delighted with your decision to consult our office, I'll refund whatever you've paid us." Assure image-conscious patients of the good company they share with countless celebrities who regularly use chiropractic care. Assure patients that "how long they decide to benefit from chiropractic is always up to them." If patients are afraid they'll be abandoned by their medical doctor, remind them that they don't have to tell their medical doctor that they're consulting your office. "I'll be happy to let your medical doctor take credit for the results you experience in our office, because you and I will know the real truth!"

Make sure the patients who are brave enough to investigate chiropractic can adequately explain and defend the decision they've made when they mention chiropractic to others. Patients who get great results in your office are often prompted to tell others, just like when we discover a special little restaurant or some other "find" we'd want to share with our friends. If we're asked a question we can't answer or if an accusation about the wisdom of our decision can't be defended, we vow not to tell others. It's just too risky. ■

ORGAN POKER

Experts say there are five ways to organize information: alphabetically, categorically, by location, time, and continuum. When these five organizing principles are used in patient education efforts, it may cause some to start with the D. D. Palmer story or the birth process (time). Others stress the relationship between various spinal levels (continuum) and the possible resulting organ damage (location). Still others direct their approach to patient education by the type of symptom the patient presents (category). Perhaps the least effective approach would be to offer the patient a glossary of terms (alphabetical) and ask if they have any questions. As a teacher, the methods you use to organize information can have a profound effect on the patient's understanding of chiropractic.

These five organizing principles make learning new information easier for our analytical minds. The absence of this order would cause information to be delivered randomly and without the proper context, making assembly directions, library card catalogs, and the information on a computer disk drive virtually impossible to find or use. The order this brings to our chaotic world, simplifies our lives and improves our productivity. Our mind's proclivity to organize, categorize, and arrange is both a blessing and a curse. It is a blessing when it serves our needs and helps us tame the world around us. It is a curse when it misrepresents reality and produces wrong conclusions. Which is often what happens to patients who enter a chiropractic office.

Most patients begin chiropractic care having long ago been

subdued by the medical model of health and healing. Besides a lifetime of living in their own bodies, using a mechanistic model to describe its function, most patients endured a grade school education that explained bodily functions, categorized by system.

I remember my sixth grade teacher, Mr. Albert Bookout, teaching the systems of the body. The first system we learned was the circulatory system. Maybe that's where your teacher started. (Over 30 years later, this emphasis on the blood system has created a generation with a fixation on heart disease, intravenous blood diseases, heart transplants, and cholesterol.) We learned the four chambers of the heart, the direction of blood flow, and used our colored pencils to show pathways of the oxygenated red blood and the blue "used" blood. Then we learned about the digestive system. Like a factory assembly line, we followed the food from the mouth and out the rectum, complete with the whispered giggles from sixth grade boys that accompanies this sort of discussion about bodily function. Eventually we got to the nervous system, which was seemingly given a less or equal importance as circulation and digestion systems!

Teaching human physiology in this compartmental way, while easy to understand, has obvious shortcomings. Among them, people see their bodies as a collection of parts, instead of as an integrated whole. It creates patients who attempt to isolate or ignore the relationship between different organs and systems. They take headache medicine, thinking the medicine has the ability to focus solely on their throbbing foreheads. They agree to have troublesome (and apparently expendable) organs removed surgically. Many view themselves as merely complicated machines with various parts whose health is considered separately, ignoring the health and function of other interrelated parts.

In the same way governments use political boundaries to define nations of the world, overlooking the fact that we all share the same planet, many patients ignore the interrelationships between all the organs and systems of the body. Every cell is in communication with every other cell. Even so, patients enter a chiropractic office thinking they have a low back problem, a sciatic nerve problem, a neck

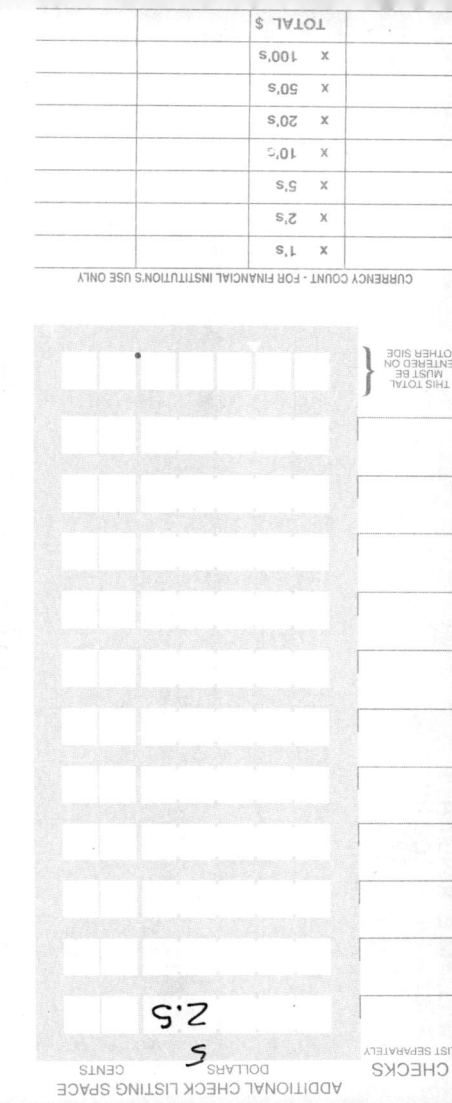

DEPOSIT TICKET

WILLIAM E. ROESCH
SUSAN EILEN ROESCH
DL N7431047 EXP. 6/97
1010 BALBOA AVE.   408-462-5904
CAPITOLA, CA   95010

BANK OF THE WEST®

DATE _____ 19 _____

DEPOSITS MAY NOT BE AVAILABLE FOR IMMEDIATE WITHDRAWAL.

SIGN HERE ONLY IF CASH RECEIVED FROM DEPOSIT

Capitola Office
3820 CAPITOLA ROAD
CAPITOLA, CALIFORNIA 95010
1-800-488-2265

☐ CASH
INCLUDING COINS ▲

List
Checks
Singly

TOTAL
ITEMS

OR TOTAL FROM REVERSE

SUB TOTAL ▲

☐ LESS CASH
RECEIVED ▲

$

⑆500⑈100015⑈ 034075135⑈

problem, or some other problem, isolated from the rest of themselves. Actually, they have a whole body problem! Remember the old fashioned Christmas tree lights? When one light burned out, it affected the entire string of lights. The Vertebral Subluxation Complex is a whole body phenomenon, too.

The preconceived notions that patients have about human physiology are formidable enemies in your attempts to explain the importance of nervous system integrity and communicate the value of a chiropractic lifestyle. These mechanistic ideas lurk in the background, out of sight, governing patient behavior. And the fact is, most patients value their spines considerably less than other organs and systems of their bodies.

In our culture, while the brain is usually recognized as the most important organ, the heart is at the top of the ladder in surgical importance. Every year, thousands of people pay for heart transplants, triple bypass operations, and invasive angioplasty. Livers and lungs score somewhat below the heart. Surgeries on colons, stomachs, throats, and hernias fall in somewhere less important than lungs and livers. In decreasing importance are spleens, gall bladders, and kidneys (after all, you have two of them). And bringing up the rear of the "organ parade" are appendixes and tonsils. For many patients, the spine and its related neurological structures are among the least important. Imagine trying to motivate a patient to understand the importance of proper spinal hygiene when they prioritize parts of their body (and the associated practitioners who deal with them) in this way!

If you accept this explanation as one of the causes of disappointing patient behavior, you also recognize the importance of overcoming it. Here are some suggestions.

1. Explain survivability needs. Many chiropractors who are successful in repositioning and reframing the importance of the nervous system, confront patients with a hierarchy of ingredients necessary to survive. "Even though you're probably going to feel hungry in a couple of hours, each of us could probably last 30 days without food. You could probably go a full week without water. And only about three minutes without a proper air supply. But, only about three seconds without a nervous system to control everything."

2. The new highway metaphor. When patients suffer from a compressive lesion and extremities go numb, it is a dramatic representation of the role of the nervous system. More subtle, more difficult, and frankly a more common problem that needs to be explained, is the far reaching affects of impaired nervous system function. "Imagine a small, bustling town located on a major state highway. The road goes through the center of town and tourists frequently stop to shop and eat at the several restaurants in town. A new interstate highway is built that goes around the town, denying it the normal circulation of traffic (subluxation). What happens to the health of that little town?"

3. The quadriplegic metaphor. To help patients better appreciate the role of the nervous system and its affect on the whole body, it may be valuable to introduce patients to this observation. "Probably one of the best ways to demonstrate the importance of a healthy nervous system is to study the affects on people who have obvious neurological deficits. The most common are paraplegics and quadriplegics. The more neurological damage there is, the shorter the lifespan; quadriplegics generally have shorter life spans than paraplegics."

Patients rarely value their spines as much as you do. (Those who do, often become chiropractors!) Until chiropractors recognize that they are working with the whole body, even though their focus is the spine and nervous system, the chances of patients properly valuing chiropractic is limited. ■

CHIROPRACTIC OVERSIMPLIFIED

There was a time, not too long ago, when doctors where put on a pedestal. They were treated as gods. "Doctor's orders" had the capacity to instill fear, or at the least, cause a patient's behavior to be at least temporarily modified. This was a time when many people barely had a high school diploma and understanding the vast complexities of the human frame were reserved for the "learned" men in white lab coats. Fortunately, that's changed. More and more of today's patients have some college under their belts, are quick to seek a third or fourth opinion, and seem willing to second guess a doctor's judgment, suing if necessary. It's amazing that in this context there are still chiropractors who are still talking about simplistic subluxations, pinched nerves, misalignments, and bones out of place!

True, fundamental chiropractic principles were reduced for countless unsophisticated generations who revered virtually any type of doctor. Fingers were pinched in foramina and the metaphor of the dead plant (organ) suffering from a water shortage (nerve interference) due to a rock (bone) pinching the hose (nerve) has been explained to millions of chiropractic patients since 1895. Besides the fact that a "pinched nerve" (compressive lesion) is a relatively rare bird (10%-15% of chiropractic cases), the real danger is that these simplistic models devalue chiropractic. Moreover, they depreciate the chiropractic skills necessary to help restore a patient's health, while minimizing the full nature and severity of the patient's problem. No wonder patients don't comply, don't bring their families in to be checked, and look to a third party to pay for their care!

Explaining the Vertebral Subluxation Complex to patients may be difficult because it takes more time and may require new communication habits. Usually we reject anything new because the fear of failure is so high. Like plunging into the buttery softness of a pair of comfortable slippers, continuing to offer patients chiropractic explanations centered around "bones out of place" and "pinched nerves" is familiar and produces the predictably inane patient acceptance so many doctors crave. However, it is vital that patients understand the full nature and severity of their problems. Try looking at it from a patient's point of view.

If you're a patient who is a member of the aforementioned generation, and you've stumbled into a chiropractic office, you probably think you have some type of spine related problem. In fact, it is the presence of some type of obvious symptom that has prompted you to seek care in the first place. Your lifetime of being exposed to the medical model of health—equating symptoms with sickness and no symptoms with health, has directed you to this health care provider. Based upon what you've been taught over the years, combined with your own often undivulged theories about health and healing, the chiropractor informs you that you have a subluxation. You've never heard of a subluxation before. Your expression prompts the chiropractor to explain further, indicating that a subluxation is when spinal bones get displaced, putting pressure on nerve roots, affecting your health. "Okay, that makes sense," you say to yourself. "Put the bone back!"

And so, that's what the doctor does. The patient hears an audible sound from the cavitation of the affected joint(s) and immediately senses progress. The symptoms may not have been instantly alleviated, but the patient is reassured by the doctor that relief usually takes a while, "After all, you've had this problem for some time. It will take time for it to heal."

So far so good.

But the real flaw in the doctor's explanation is just around the corner. Since (whether the doctor likes it or not) the patient was self-directed to the office because of recognizable symptoms, he or she will most likely use this same yardstick to measure the need for continued care. Under the simplistic subluxation model, with the "bone back in place" and the "pinched nerve" no longer pinching and producing symptoms, patients have not only fulfilled their own medical model of appropriate treatment, they have apparently fulfilled the chiropractor's model as well! Whether the patient stays for two visits or 12 visits or however long a third party will pay the way, the patient has apparently recovered, but became a victim in the process. Besides having their myopic view of chiropractic affirmed, patients are likely to make poor decisions about their health and misread the doctor's overtures for continue chiropractic care on a nonsymptomatic basis. Because of the limited "subluxation" explanation, the doctor/patient relationship often degenerates into a tragic lose/lose confrontation.

When you take the initiative to explain the five components of the Vertebral Subluxation Complex, using appropriate metaphors to explain the concepts of motion/position of spinal bones, facilitative/compressive lesions, muscle and soft tissues damage, and the resulting degenerative changes from neglect, you raise a patient's esteem for you and your profession. Happily, this often results in more respect, better compliance, and a new enthusiasm for chiropractic. Again, from a patient's point of view, here are some ways to position these five components in a patient's mind for better understanding:

1. Spinal Kinesiopathology. We know that spinal bones can lose their normal motion or position. This can occur from trauma, tension, or toxins. A majority of the profession seems to agree that chiropractic plays a role in helping to restore biomechanical function to the spine. This usually takes the form of some type of specific chiropractic adjustment, adding motion to hypomobile joints by the introduction of appropriate forces along malfunctioning joint planes. There seems to be more disagreement about *how* this is done, than *why* it is done.

This is the unique domain of chiropractic doctors and the most obvious aspect of a patient's chiropractic experience. They get adjusted. Bones are moved. It sets in motion (or reduces) other physiologic responses. Patients sense something is happening to them. Based upon appropriate tableside manners, the skills necessary to move the right bones, the right amount, can produce respect and even awe.

The patient point: This is what chiropractors do to help patients.

2. Neuropathophysiology. This component is essential to explain to patients because it shows how aberrant spinal biomechanics produce a whole body response due to the direct affect of the nervous system. Here, it is absolutely critical that patients understand the facilitative lesion; the rubbing, stretching, twisting, or irritation of delicate nerve tissue. If you want patients to understand the value of nonsymptomatic chiropractic care, avoid the temptation to focus on the compressive lesion!

The facilitative lesion is more subtle. Symptoms aren't always obvious. This is why many patients experience relief or improvement with health problems that aren't usually thought of as "back problems." This is why, if you want to be your best, you want to be checked even on a nonsymptomatic basis. With this knowledge, you'd want to have your loved ones checked too.

The patient point: Chiropractic care can have positive affects throughout the body.

3. Myopathology. Muscles that support the spine are involved, becoming flaccid and weakening or becoming tight, going into spasm. Scar tissue forms in these malfunctioning muscles, changing their elasticity. These muscles play an important part in the recovery process and can take a long time to retrain and offer bilateral stability. "How long would it take you to bulk up and acquire enough muscle to become a weight lifter?" It takes time to strengthen the muscles that support your spine too.

The patient point: It's going to take more than just a couple of adjustments.

4. Histopathology. Discs, ligaments, cartilage, and other soft tissues have a very poor blood supply. In fact, these tissues depend heavily upon the pumping action of joint fluids to supply nutrients and express waste products. When this pumping action is impaired, these critical soft tissues don't heal with the speed today's patient wants or expects. Denying patients access to this critical information because it's new, or you think patients don't want to know, sets yourself up for disappointment later when patients make inappropriate or shortsighted decisions about their health.

The patient point: It's going to take a long time to heal.

5. Pathophysiology. Over time, if the problem is neglected, the body will attempt to splint or stabilize the injured joint, like mending a broken bone. First, a thickening of adjacent bone surfaces, then a lipping effect, bone spurs, and ultimately fusion. This and other degenerative changes affect the spine and other organs and tissues throughout the body which are deprived of normal nerve supply.

The patient point: If you neglect your problem it will get worse.

Patients who are fed the pabulum of "bones pinching nerves" are shortchanged. They are given merely a thumbnail sketch of their problem, so they don't see the significance of chiropractic care. It's like telling someone that the consequences of attempting to breathe underwater will merely fill their lungs with water. It's true, but there's more to it! Same with subluxations. ■

PUSHING OR PULLING?

My early interest in electronics came in the early 1960s, soon after the widespread availability of the transistor. I recall that transistors came in two basic designs, either a PNP or a NPN. I no longer remember the significance of these two differences or what the initials stand for, but I do remember the fascination I had about how those tiny devices could amplify an electrical signal. The circuits for many amplifiers were referred to as "push-pull" designs. Apparently, the way the voltages were manipulated, they were "pushed" and then "pulled" into a new, louder form. Are you pushing patient education upon patients, or are you pulling them towards your knowledge and understanding?

With amazing regularity, one of the car dealerships in town will ask potential customers to "push, pull, or drag" their old cars to the lot so they can trade it in for enormous savings on a new car. In other words, do whatever it takes to get the old car to our lot and get a good deal. I suppose if you needed a new car, you'd get behind your old clunker and push it to the dealership. Same as if you were to run out of gas 50 feet from the pump. Like pushing patient education upon a new patient, pushing is hard work! And like the debilitated car, most patients don't particularly appreciate your efforts. Pushing horses to a watering hole to drink, or pushing patients towards a greater understanding of true health, is rarely successful. In fact, force-feeding patient education (or anything else), can appear quite suspicious to a patient. They search for your motives and question the reasons for your apparent interest in their understanding. Some patients "push back" by consciously ignoring your furtive attempts.

Like the wild-eyed street corner evangelist, patients often reject direct patient education overtures when they are pushed upon them. We'll avoid the street corner or deride the inappropriate style being used. Like enough coats of paint on a do-it-yourself project at home, it's easy to think that with just enough videos, posters, brochures, and lectures, your well-intentioned patient education message will "take" and patients will become grateful students, hanging on your every word. This is probably more rare than street corner conversions at the hands of a Bible thumping preacher!

How do you make the "pull" of patient education so compelling that patients ask great questions, appreciate your answers, and want to know even more?

1. Don't care too much. With the countless seminars devoted to the "love concept" in chiropractic and the value of unconditionally loving each patient, this suggestion may seem difficult to accept. However, one of the common mistakes some of the most dedicated chiropractors make is the way they demonstrate their caring.

These doctors have seen countless clinical examples of patients who delayed or discontinued care, resulting in needless suffering and, later, irreversible damage. This tremendous waste causes many doctors to suggest preventive strategies to help patients avoid unnecessary pain and suffering. While a doctor's selfless interest is understandable, patients are often suspicious of anyone, particularly someone with a financial interest, who seems inordinately interested in their behavior beyond the obvious. Worse, by smothering the patient by strongly suggesting a specific course of action, when the eventual recovery results, the doctor "steals" the satisfaction from a patient for having made the correct decision! In other words, your attempts to control patient behavior can backfire, producing a patient who resents the apparent dependence they have, or had, on you. So while they got the outcome they wanted, they didn't get the commensurate emotional satisfaction usually due someone whose independent decision results in good fortune.

An interesting paradox occurs when you lay out the realities of a patient's presenting complaints and the consequences of the various choices before them, and assume an "I-don't-care-what-you-do-because-it's-your-life" attitude, compliance and interest in chiropractic grows. Apparently, releasing control (which you don't really have anyway!) creates more interest, more confidence in you, and draws a patient closer. Your objectivity, and the confidence it projects, can magnetize patients to want more, know more, and strengthen their resolve.

This is the "tough love" approach. It's because you really care, that you should resist the temptation to rush in and solve their problems, turning yourself into a hero in the process. Besides giving the credit for healing to the patient's body, make sure you allow the patient the opportunity to take credit for their decision to comply with your recommendations.

2. Ask good questions. Countless chiropractors attempt to foist the chiropractic approach onto patients, instead of pulling the patients up to their level. They push brochures, videos, and messages interspersed among music selections emitting from speakers in the reception room ceiling. Many doctors tire of this constant pushing, telling the D.D. Palmer story for the billionth time, pinching the patient's finger in the foramina of an anatomical model, and taking criticism from patients who don't want to watch a "propaganda-filled" video. And yet, conventional wisdom suggests that the better patients understand chiropractic, the more likely they are to make appropriate decisions about their health. Who said force-feeding patients your chiropractic dogma actually educates patients and changes their behavior? Has it worked so far?

I remember getting an occasional spanking as a child. This was before it wasn't politically correct to actually punish a child to instill discipline. I remember my mom saying, "This is going to hurt me a whole lot more than it's going to hurt you." At the time, I didn't understand how that could be, since she used a wooden spoon on my rear end. Now, as a parent, I understand perfectly. Even as doctors tire of telling the same story over and over again, tap dancing in front of the X-ray view box, and coercing staff members to use the phone to badger wayward patients who opt not to follow recommendations, they justify their burden as being in the best interests of the patient. Really?

What countless patients are saying when they vote with their feet, by ignoring or discontinuing your care recommendations is, "Chiropractic is unnecessary because I feel fine." "I value (my car payments, dinners out, vacation, etc.) more than my health." "I got what I wanted." "I can't justify the expense any more." "I didn't get it." Instead of finding out what would make chiropractic relevant to each patient, it must be easier to pummel them with health tracts and well-intentioned reminders to maintain a visit schedule they don't want or understand.

The only way to make chiropractic relevant for patients is to ask questions. "What do you hope to do better or enjoy more when you regain your health?" "Why are you here today?" "What would it take to encourage you to adopt some type of on-going maintenance care?" These and similar questions help give patients an opportunity to reveal their concerns and divulge issues that can help you tailor your educational protocol. A one-size-fits-all patient education regime, doesn't.

An airplane rises because the shape of the wing creates low pressure above it as it moves through the air. This low pressure can be so powerful, it can lift tons of aluminum, passengers, and baggage. The airplane is literally pulled up into the sky by this partial vacuum above its wings. Same with patients. Patients can be drawn, or pulled towards you (and chiropractic) by asking questions that cause a vacuum to be produced. "How do you explain cancer?" "How do you explain spontaneous remission?" "How do you explain how your body knows to deposit calcium at the site of a broken bone?" "Why do some people 'catch' a cold and others in the same office don't? What controls that?" "How does the headache medicine know to go to the head?" You create a vacuum by asking questions that patients find difficult or impossible to answer, based upon their incorrect notions of how the body functions. Coming up empty-handed, or revealing a childish or simplistic answer to questions like these, creates an uneasiness and ambiguity makes most people uncomfortable. Suddenly, they're interested.

Don't rush in!

Avoid the temptation to rush in for the kill. Let the pressure mount. Perhaps ask even more questions. At some point, maybe the next visit, the seeds you've planted will start to sprout, spawning a sincere interest in the form of a brilliant question that, for you, will make showing up at the office the joy it should be. Even after using every tool, every technique, asking every question, and doing everything you can think of, there will be patients who still don't want to know about your philosophy or unique perspective. It's okay. Help them with what they want, and continue your search for patients who *are* interested.

While pushing patient education upon a patient can be gratifying because it makes you feel like you're in control, it is actually the patient who is at the helm. Push if you want, but pulling is more fun—and probably a lot more effective. ■

SPINAL FLOSSING

It still astounds me that so many chiropractors who regularly get adjusted on a "wellness" or nonsymptomatic basis, are quick to denounce the value of similar care for their patients. True, succumbing to the notion that obvious symptoms must be present to justify the need for an adjustment is congruent with "accepted" mainstream medical approaches to health care. The only problem is, the mainstream medical community is facing epidemic health problems which are lifestyle induced and whose symptoms only appear at the latest and most problematical stages, such as hypertension, cancer, arteriosclerosis, and a host of immune deficiency diseases. Health problems whose first and most obvious symptoms are often death!

So much for conventional mainstream thinking.

Not long ago I visited my dentist, or more accurately, my dental hygienist. It's a client relationship going on 17 years. I always look forward to meeting with Jean and catching up on the previous nine months. No talk about aches or pains. No whining. When you share similar values, the relationship is deeper, more fulfilling, and more significant. Symptoms are boring. "How's the family?" "Did you get to Bermuda like you were planning?" Client relationships are very different from patient relationships.

After catching up on the latest goings on, she went to work. After a couple of minutes, and with her instruments still in my mouth I asked her "Sowaa'ste oost 'trustin pooort offyerjab?"

Since you went to chiropractic college and not to dental assisting school, you probably wouldn't have been able to understand my question. But she deciphered it perfectly. She said, "Well, the most frustrating part of my job is seeing the way people care for their teeth and gums and knowing that if they don't make a change, they're going to lose their teeth in 10 or 20 years. The most difficult part is trying to figure out what to say or do to get patients to change their behavior."

Sound familiar?

Imagine the challenge a dentist or hygienist faces when they beg, cajole, grovel, plead, and implore patients to floss their teeth. Try to comprehend the frustration of just getting patients to brush their teeth regularly. But all too many patients refuse to perform these simple, inexpensive, yet highly-effective self-care procedures. **Compare the investment of time and energy needed to conduct these simple procedures at home, with what you're asking your patients to do, by swinging by your office after work once or twice a month, to sit in a crowded reception room and drop 30 bucks for a non-symptomatic wellness visit!**

Many of your patients are more conscientious about the maintenance of their automobiles than their own bodies—because they value their cars more than they do themselves. Because they value the image their cars project about them more than themselves. Because they value the investment they made in their cars more than themselves. Because their friends can see their cars, but can't see their spine. Because they understand their cars, more obviously depend upon their cars, and associate their cars with feelings of power and control more than their own bodies! In their cars they control hundreds of horses. In their bodies they are victims, warding off infections, invasions of germs, and fight a losing battle to control their weight. Their cars help them feel good. Their bodies are associated with pain.

Any wonder patients who drive expensive cars can't seem to "afford" maintenance chiropractic care?

Overcoming this predisposition is difficult, maybe impossible. Does that mean you shouldn't try? Of course you should. And, you probably have tried in the past. (Remember, this is the most frustrating part of chiropractic!) But, if your past efforts have not produced the results you desire, perhaps you should try some new strategies.

Patient education: At the risk of becoming a broken record, patient education is crucial if you are to ever change these default patient beliefs and health habits. Patient education is a lot more than a dynamic report of findings and pantomiming like the TV weatherman in front of the X-ray view box! How about making your patient education relevant to the patient's occupation? How about using lots of metaphors and models? How about asking questions that reveal the patient's belief system? How about exploiting every visit and every opportunity to expand the patient's knowledge? How about it?

Visit mnemonic: Battery companies have chosen the two times a year when we change our clocks from and to daylight savings time as a reminder to change the batteries in our smoke detectors. Not only does this sell a lot of batteries, it fulfills an important public service by reminding everyone of the importance of maintaining their smoke detectors. It's probably saved countless lives. What are you doing to encourage patients to return to your office with some type of regularity? Payday? First of the month? Quarterly? New Year's resolution? Birthday? Anniversary of the first chiropractic adjustment? Anniversary of *their* first chiropractic adjustment?

What would it take: All too often doctors regurgitate a pre-packaged care plan that they expect patients to follow without question. Why not find out what it would take to convince a patient to continue with some type of regular wellness plan? Ask patients what it would take to motivate them to continue showing up once or twice a week/month, or whatever your idea of maintenance care is? "What could we do to make some type of preventive care attractive to you with your busy schedule?" "Based upon your care so far, how often do you sense you should be coming in for a maintenance visit? What would we need to do to make that visit frequency affordable?" Instead of playing coy, cut to the chase. What would the patient be willing to go for? Something's better than nothing!

Create a place for wellness patients. More often then you'll ever know, patients who have been under care in the past and want a "tune-up", drive past your office. Many count the number of cars in your parking lot and reach the conclusion that they don't have time to stop. For these patients, it may not be the monetary cost of your care, it's the amount of time it takes to *get* care. What is so innocuous about this phenomenon, is that you don't know when it's happening—you don't have a traffic counter laid across the road out front to count inactive patients as they pass by! Pick a day of the week or the month and reserve it for wellness patients. Let them know that on that day you promise to see patients in less than XX minutes or the visit is free. Remove the time barrier as an excuse for patients to avoid remaining under care.

"How can I help you today?" Patients have spent their entire lives judging their health by the presence or absence of symptoms. Retraining patients on this most critical issue requires constant attention. Asking patients on each visit why they are in your office and what they want you to do, is a powerful way to make your point. When patients whine about an ache or pain, remind them of your true mission. When patients seem surprised by your question, remind them that the first symptom of lifestyle induced diseases such as cancer and hypertension, is death. Reframe patients' symptoms so they become more interested in structure and function and less consumed by their symptoms.

What is it that prompts one patient to religiously floss his or her teeth, and another to ignore this inexpensive self-care procedure? What is it that prompts one person to compulsively wash and vacuum his or her car, while others drive around town in a rolling rat hole? What is it that persuades one person to consistently wear a seat belt, and another to taunt Newtonian physics? Birth order? Awareness? Education? Peer pressure? Self-esteem?

It may be that the seemingly most desirable health attitudes are formed at an early age. How did your mom react to little health emergencies when you were growing up? How clean did you have to keep your room? Did you live in a "treat the symptoms" environment or a "preventive" environment? How important was self-discipline in your family?

Certainly each doctor has a responsibility to expand a patient's knowledge and appreciation of true health. And of course, every doctor has the duty to help prevent that which they treat. And certainly, every doctor has the obligation to empower a patient with appropriate information and self-care procedures. But, pushing too hard flies in the face of the words of a famous philosopher, Popeye, the Sailor Man who always said, "I y'am what I y'am." Which is why Popeye was a sailor, and you're a doctor. ■

OUT OF CONTROL

In our misguided efforts to control our lives, we attempt to force our narrow perspectives onto others. Many use threats, coercion, position, and fear to get people, patients, staff members, etc. to perform. Third parties, such as insurance companies and managed care organizations base their control schemes (or derivations of these techniques) on doctors. Besides revealing a basic mistrust for others, this style of management costs individual practitioners thousands of dollars every month! Since chiropractors, even the best intentioned, never receive an invoice for the amounts their controlling strategies cost them, it is often difficult to recognize, much less change.

Ironically, at the very moment chiropractic proves itself to new patients, who then, based upon their medical model of health, attempt to disengage from the practice, countless doctors spoil a perfectly good patient relationship. The pressure is subtle at first as a patient misses scheduled appointments or doesn't seem to take the need for continued care as seriously as the doctor. Phone calls, postcards and other "reminders" are often used to prompt patients to stay on the straight and narrow. Imagine how these pathetic attempts must seem to a patient who is experiencing pain-free living for the first time in years! Why continue taking aspirin if your headache is gone?

If low-force control schemes don't produce appropriately docile patients to continue their care on a non-symptomatic basis, the larger artillery is brought out. Now, wayward patients are petitioned by only half-convincing staff members who deploy every scripted means possible to cajole a patient to return to the office. "Uh... the doctor has found something on your X-rays he needs to discuss with you..."

Do these and other equally manipulative scripts prompt patients to return to the office? Some actually seem to work. While countless doctors rationalize that they're simply looking out for the best interests of the patient, they are unknowingly committing a cardinal sin.

It might not be a confrontive phone call. Sometimes it's a letter, still trying to convince the patient of the value of continued care. Regardless of the medium, patients often perceive these attempts as a form of scolding. Rarely do these attempts succeed in producing anything more than banishing the patient from your office. Has any heavy-handed recall effort produced a patient who finally got the "big idea" and signed up for lifetime chiropractic care? Ever?

Certainly this is an issue of timing, but perhaps more insidious is the paternalistic notion that prompts doctors to feel compelled to look out after these poor patients because "they know not what they do." While the most cynical inside (and outside) the profession believe that trying to keep patients continuing care on a non-symptomatic basis is financially driven, I don't think so. It's almost always attempted out of total devotion and caring for the patient. After all, you can't accurately judge one's health by whether or not there are symptoms. So, the motive may be pure, but the technique stinks.

When patients leave, it's almost like being turned down for the prom. When patients leave, it's like no one wanting to come to our party. When patients leave, it's like being the last one chosen for the softball team. When patients leave, it's easy to take the rejection personally. Attempting to make up for lost opportunities, inadequate patient explanations, or ineptly handled patient education efforts by ramming continued chiropractic down their throats, when they're "feeling fine," produces counterproductive results.

The fact is, very few patients ever really "get it." Over the years, there are only a handful of doctors I've met who have the ability to lead their patients to a higher level of understanding about health and healing. Interestingly, these are the same doctors who produce countless disciples willing to forsake other career paths to become chiropractors themselves. **If you're not regularly inspiring patients to go to chiropractic college, I can almost guarantee you're not connecting with your patients on more than a superficial, pain relief-only level.**

If you're dissatisfied with treating an endless stream of patients who don't understand, don't respect what you do, don't refer their friends and families, and don't adopt a chiropractic lifestyle, here are some specific action steps you might want to consider.

Set a good example. First of all, doctors who are truly effective in transforming patient beliefs and understanding about health are interesting doctors. The personal standards they set for themselves and expect from their staff are legendary. Their lives are living testimonials to a preoccupation with "cause." So you won't find them in co-dependent relationships with spouses or staff members. Some patients may take advantage of them because they wear their hearts on their sleeves, but most patients find their openness and vulnerability attractive. They are principled, disciplined, and humble enough to recognize the high calling of serving others. Interestingly, these character issues are rarely the subject of weekend practice building seminars.

Clarify your beliefs. It's difficult to muster the requisite passion if your belief system is muddy, or too easily susceptible to the whims of patients, circumstances, or financial pressures. A wise man once observed that "people don't steal because they are poor, they are poor because they steal." How true. To become truly powerful and influential with your patients you must clarify your position. The only way to go boldly and make decisions swiftly is to know your purpose. The only way to inspire confidence in others, is to have confidence in yourself. These are the qualities of true leadership. They are not obtained by watching television. They are not secured by squandering precious time with sports scores and other inconsequential diversions. Remember Jesus' 40 days in the wilderness? Perhaps you need to spend some time alone, contemplating all this. Why not reserve 20 minutes every morning? Get reacquainted with yourself. What do you believe? What do you stand for? Develop and clarify a point of view!

Confront patients. I'm not suggesting the heavy-handed techniques mentioned above! The doctors who come to mind who have been so successful in inspiring others, are as watchful as a hawk. They are masters at asking questions. Questions clarify. When they see a patient exhibiting signs of fuzzy logic or reaching incorrect conclusions, they simply ask, "So why do you think that is?" With Trojan Horse stealth, they open the eyes of their patients and reveal new ways of thinking—and behavior by helping patients question the status quo. More importantly, they recognize the limitations of a brief, three-times-a-week encounter. Instead of aiming for the bleachers, or going for the long bomb, they lower their sights to a more realistic level. Their ability to establish rapport and assume a non-judgmental posture gives patients confidence to ask questions and try out new ideas about their health. These doctors recognize that incremental change is less traumatic and longer lasting.

Become outspoken. Needless to say, these doctors are fearless communicators. Because they are very clear in what they believe, they are willing to passionately deliver their message. Their dogmatic stance may make some observers uncomfortable. Better to stand behind an idea or belief 100%, even if unpopular, than to blunt one's impact by looking for political correctness. The willingness to champion your point of view is directly related to your confidence and belief. The only way to gain this confidence is to voice your opinions and submit your ideas to the sharpening agent of public exposure. Keeping your perspectives to yourself, even if they are correct, effective, or empowering for you, never have the "legs" to stand on their own without the exposure to critical review. While it may be challenging to justify and defend your perspective, it is only in the testing, defending, and advocating of your opinions that they can be sufficiently strong and sharply defined to be first, understandable, then attractive, and then embraced by others.

The fact is, doctors can't control patients. It's a myth. Just try to control the behavior of someone you barely know, only rarely see, and depend upon for a paycheck! A more realistic strategy might be to control yourself. ■

PREP SCHOOL

My very first job was selling blackberries door to door to those wanting to bake pies but not endure the thorns and hot sun. My second job was mowing lawns in my neighborhood using my Dad's old rotary lawn mower. Paper routes. Washing dishes at a local restaurant. Shelving books at the public library. Each of us has an early job history that has probably never shown up on a resume, but affects the way we each work today. Which is why so many student doctors become indentured servants to established doctors.

Many students came to chiropractic because they saw it as a chance to make a lot of money, especially in the rollicking days of the 1980s. All too many chiropractic college professors lament about the number of students who didn't receive their first chiropractic adjustment until after arriving at school. "We've got an entire generation of students who got involved in chiropractic for the wrong reason," they sigh, looking wistfully upward.

Is this where the chiropractic poverty complex gets rooted, by chiropractic college teachers who scorn money and its implications? Teachers who find the real world unfamiliar and their skills ignored by paying customers, retreat to the institution that bred them, infecting others. Students who find they must withstand the entrepreneurial pressures of those who conduct management seminars for the optimism and leadership they crave, are seduced into financially crippling contracts. A profession that seeks acceptance and has such a low self-image looks to insurance companies, HMOs, hospitals, and the federal government for validation. New graduates who have paid tuition fees based upon a different time in chiropractic, leave with a choice-reducing debt around their necks. It seems their only solution is to prostrate themselves in front of field doctors and beg for the opportunity to conduct exams, process X-rays, and wash the doctor's car.

As a cruel test, all too many states schedule their board examinations a week or two *before* the graduation dates of most chiropractic colleges. Insecure doctors living in a zero-sum mentality (your success diminishes my success) or who have adopted a scarcity outlook (there are only so many patients and I want my share), have become examination board members and have created this barrier in the hopes of discouraging new doctors from considering their particular state or locality.

I guess it's worked so far...

Having an existing practitioner as a mentor is a good thing. But while waiting for your license there are other things you can do that could be even more profitable and help you successfully launch your new practice. If I was cooling my heels after enduring a long commencement exercise and storing my cap and gown, here are some things I'd do:

1. Tour lots of practices. Some say imitation is the sincerest form of flattery. I agree. It's valuable to see what works (and doesn't work) in other practices. You'll still make some mistakes, but you'll avoid some, too.

Work with your alumni association, technique club, or with a few of the "movers and shakers" in the chiropractic association or society of the state in which you want to practice. Get the names of those who use a similar technique or went to the same college, and ask to spend a day touring their practice and going on rounds. Explain your situation. Buy them lunch and pick their brains. "What would you do if you were just starting practice today?" "How did you get your first 10 patients?" "What's the most important aspect of the doctor/patient relationship?" "How do you handle skeptical patients?"

As long as you ask questions, keep your own opinions to yourself, and try to honestly see the wisdom of their point of view, you'll learn a lot. This will be information you won't find in a book, a tape, or a seminar. Keep a log or a journal. Tour 20, 30, 50, or more offices.

2. Conduct patient focus groups. Maybe in conjunction with your office tours you can earn a few bucks by conducting a patient focus group for the field doctor.

Arrange to meet five or six patients for lunch at a nearby restaurant. Ask them questions about what they like and don't like about the practice, the procedures, the staff, the parking; that sort of thing. Explain to the patients that you'll keep their names confidential, but your job is to uncover ways the office can offer better service to its patients.

The information you uncover for the doctor will be invaluable. Besides picking up some cash on top of the expense of the meals, you'll be learning incredible insights about how today's real live patients think and act. You'll see chiropractic practice entirely different, and I can guarantee your own practice will be more relevant, more attractive, and more successful.

3. Seek public speaking opportunities. It is said that those who can't, teach. Since you can't practice—yet, you might as well teach!

Since the caliber of your communication skills are an accurate indicator of your success as a chiropractor, confront your fears. Put your understanding of chiropractic to the test by speaking to any group looking for a speaker. Check with your chamber of commerce, toastmaster group, or the editor of the suburban weekly newspapers. Find out who needs a speaker.

If this suggestion makes you uncomfortable, you are the perfect candidate for this exercise. Your ability to articulate your philosophy, your treatment style, and describe the mythical practice of your dreams can help assure it becomes a reality. Perhaps only without a practice of your own can you most effectively "sell" chiropractic without worrying about the perception that you're out soliciting patients.

4. Become a patient education specialist. This is what I want to do someday! Find a busy field doctor who recognizes the value of educated patients, but doesn't have the time or systems to make it happen. Become the "new patient advocate." Design and implement a comprehensive patient education strategy.

Prepare patients for every office function and be the new patient's liaison in the office. Lay the groundwork for the patient's report of findings. Clean up and organize the admitting paperwork, patient policy handouts, and other documents. Conduct patient lectures, seminars, and workshops. Experiment with different metaphors and communication devices to help convey the chiropractic message.

You want to get paid for doing this? Remind the treating doctor that there is a CPT code for patient education (99071). Perhaps you can split this fee with the office and maybe pick up an additional fee based upon your ability to increase the patient visit average or case fee average. Be creative. It may be minimum wage, but you'll be in an office acquiring a skill that may be one of the most important aspects of practice in the 1990s.

5. Conduct neighborhood surveys. I had to throw this one in, because I've heard how effective it can be, if done properly. It's a twist on the focus group idea mentioned earlier. Tour the area in which you are intending to open your practice and go door to door asking questions.

Remember, while your practice may be nine months away, most patients wait even longer before garnering the courage to consult a chiropractic office. So don't be afraid of planting "seeds" when you have no practice with which to harvest them.

Ask questions about the practicalities of opening an office in the area, such as traffic patterns, parking problems, or other practical matters. Ask about their experiences with chiropractors in the past. What are some of the qualities they'd look for in a chiropractor. That sort of thing. Take notes! Buy a mailing list and use it to code who you've talked to and their openness to your survey. Send them a follow-up "thank you" card! Later invite them to your open house. Get the picture?

Will there be people who will slam their door in your face? Of course. Will there be dogs waiting to chew on your leg? Probably. Will there be people with a negative chiropractic experience and choose you to do a little venting? Sure. Mark Victor Hanson has the perfect antidote. You simply say to yourself, "Next!" and move on.

Starting a practice is not easy. Much of the difficulty arises from one's expectations not meeting reality. Add to this the fear of rejection and you have a formula that paralyzes many new graduates. Welcome. You've just taken the first pop quiz at the School of Hard Knocks! ∎

ENTER TO LEARN HOW

As each chiropractic college disgorges a new crop of chiropractors prepared to face licensing boards, students suddenly turn their attention from learning how to pass the board, to the acquisition of the skills necessary to run a practice. Many look for shortcuts or a recipe book that can show them how to successfully run a small business. Like searching for "an old test," these new doctors seem more interested in doing things right, than doing the right things. This misplaced allegiance to a protocol, a procedure, a script, or a form is understandable, given the dogma and prejudice surrounding the choosing of an adjusting technique.

There is an undeniable smell of fear on the breath of these new graduates. Some, who come to chiropractic as second careers, seem more confident. They appear to be more attuned to the concepts of supply and demand, customer service, and that the notion of profit is an essential ingredient to survival. Unfortunately, the fear that many graduates lacking real-world experience frequently encounter, is well-founded. Little of the experience gleaned in chiropractic college resembles the reality of private practice enough to produce the confidence necessary to exchange their valuable skills in a profitable manner!

So, while chiropractic colleges continue to churn out diplomaed graduates who are generally successful in passing state boards, they have played a cruel trick, and in the process created a market for entrepreneurial forces and a parasitic "management" industry that preys on those tasked with carrying the chiropractic torch for its second hundred years.

As the division and backbiting plaguing chiropractic continues at perhaps a greater intensity than ever before, this profession loses valuable time and opportunities for advancement. When medical doctors disagree about a procedure or diagnosis, they don't denigrate their fellow doctors. But when disagreements arise in chiropractic, many of the least secure doctors seem quick to put down or discredit someone with a different viewpoint. Attempting to validate oneself by invalidating others is an old remedy.

If only it were more successful.

When the pioneers were attacked while traveling in hostile territory, they circled their wagons. They defended themselves by shooting at the marauding Indians or bandits from behind their temporary fortress. When chiropractic is assailed, many chiropractors seem inclined to use the occasion to shoot at each other from within the circled wagons! The target in their cross hairs either uses an "experimental" technique, only takes two minutes with a patient, is an insurance "whore," or graduated from the "wrong" chiropractic college. Meanwhile, the enemy sets fire to the wagons and rapes the womenfolk.

Apparently one of the most important objectives for new doctors (second to actually graduating), is choosing the right adjusting technique. As students walk down the halls past the bulletin boards of the "approved" technique clubs, there are subtle pressures to attend the next meeting, which will feature a presentation from the visiting entrepreneurial technique instructor. As students choose their weapons in the fight against abnormal spinal biomechanics, they are quickly labeled, categorized, and often the target of disparaging terms of endearment. The seeds of suspicion, bias, and even bigotry within the profession get planted here. In increasingly subtle and destructive ways, the importance of "why" you adjust is replaced by an inordinate focus on "how" you adjust.

No wonder patients who don't respond to your adjusting style are rarely referred to another chiropractor with an entirely different approach: they're the enemy. In fact, "the profession would be much better off if it just weren't for those chiropractors who do such and such!"

Perhaps worse than the bias against various adjusting techniques or the reputation assigned by attending a particular chiropractic college, is the horrendous debt doctors graduate with. This turns graduating doctors into slaves in more direct ways than any managed care scheme!

The Old Testament addresses this issue in the book of *Proverbs* quite clearly. Besides several admonitions not to co-sign a loan, many proverbs remind us how the borrower becomes beholden to the lender and how the lender controls the borrower. If you need a textbook example of this, just look to any chiropractic college.

At a time when more and more doctors are battling managed care (which often reimburses 50 cents or less on the dollar), and the realization that most patients with $1000 deductibles can't afford to pay $50 office visits three times a week, many offices are lowering their fees. No one likes to talk about it because it suggests a flawed ability to "confront" or some other shortcoming. Meanwhile, chiropractic colleges continue to escalate the cost of their tuition, as if patients with $100 deductibles were still flocking to free spinal exams. The result is frantic doctors with a burden to produce an income at all costs.

New graduates are handicapped in their pursuit of profitably exchanging their services by an incredible lack of patient communication training. Bent on producing graduates with the best percentage of being able to pass the national board examination, little focus is given to tableside manners, office protocol, report of findings, patient education, and the communication skills essential for effective doctor/patient relationships. Even the college clinic sanctions a pain-relief-only perspective, counting patient visits only, and giving little credit or incentive to create and nurture a long-term patient relationship! So, many doctors emerge from chiropractic college with the technical skills necessary to move bones and restore the patient's inborn recuperative abilities, but increasingly are unable to form coherent sentences, produce persuasive arguments, or bond with patients—essential skills for survival in the post-insurance era.

The wisest new doctors recognize the shortcomings of their education and seek assistance from a variety of seminars, management programs, and entrepreneurial organizations. The fact that they are even aware of the importance of these skills, suggests that they have a head start on achieving the satisfaction and fulfillment they sought when choosing chiropractic as a career. It is the huge contingent of "technogeeks" who lack chiropractic philosophy (because it's not politically correct to teach it on campus), and who can't communicate with intelligence and passion, who represent the greatest threat to the survival of chiropractic. Stripping away all else to the exclusion of diagnosis and orthopedic functions, creates uncompassionate spine mechanics, not the vitalistic healers that today's health care consumer seems to be seeking. Instead, we have the cold, distant analytical clinicians that were previously reserved for the inner workings of a hospital. The solution?

1. How about some personality testing upon acceptance at chiropractic college? No need to exclude shy, personality-challenged students, but at least give them the lead time and necessary warnings that actual practice will be especially difficult for them.

2. Add public speaking courses and communication skills to each doctor's course load. If colleges were truly interested in producing effective, successful chiropractors, they would insist on graduating individuals who can form complete sentences, whether one on one, or in front of a group.

3. Teach the latest patient education protocols on campus. In most college clinics, patient education is relegated to a brief report of findings and some tap-dancing in front of an X-ray view box. If you're care is virtually free at the student clinic, perhaps that's all it takes. But not in the real world.

4. Reward alumni who are willing to take in new graduates. Create some type of incentive for field doctors who have been out on their own for five years or so, to take a graduating student under their wings. Organize a mentoring program.

5. Honor graduating students who are able to attain the highest retention levels with patients at the student clinic. Too many colleges honor graduating students for the highest GPA, technique awards, and other qualifications that do little to assure success in the real world.

6. Instead of the rhythm-breaking and numbing detail required at the college clinic, create an "advanced" clinic program where office visits are more like the time and treatment protocol of private practice.

Just as field doctors must adapt to changes in insurance reimbursement, managed care rears its ugly head, and the population increasingly seeks non-drug and non-surgical solutions, so too must chiropractic colleges adapt. The next generation of chiropractors must be ready to protect the chiropractic idea, and not be hampered by huge debts, crippled communication skills, or unrealistic expectations. ∎

denial@chiropractic.now

Increasingly, I'm encountering doctors so entrenched in their 1986 view of chiropractic that it's difficult to communicate with them. Like Rip Van Winkle, waking up from a 20 year sleep, these doctors have lost touch with the not so subtle shift that is occurring, not just in chiropractic, but in our culture. Perhaps if the changes sweeping the profession had to do with some startlingly new insight into biomechanics or revelations about the healing process, it would be easier for these doctors to assimilate. Instead, the changes foisted upon them has to do with patient issues of time, money, value, perception, compliance, and professional image—topics that are ostensibly missing from the chiropractic journals that clutter the corner of these same doctors desks!

These societal changes require adaptation and integration on a scale that can be quite challenging for doctors who have nursed on juicy insurance policies and the lump sums of personal injury awards. Naturally, the first response is predictable.

The denial stage. Because the implications of the changing practice environment run counter to the established world view of the doctor, many doctors first reject the new reality. You can hear them boasting to others how they "aren't participating in the recession." Or, they're signing up for every managed care organization they can, thinking it's merely a different form of insurance. At this stage, the primary motive is to maintain the status quo. Looking for something to focus their eyes on in the distance to avoid a seasick feeling, many become lost, searching for the latest treatment codes, still whipping the insurance horse, that lies moaning on the ground.

The anger stage. Then, doctors become indignant! They seem to think that just because virtually all the latest research has been pro chiropractic, that patients (money, prestige, and respect) should automatically flow towards their practice. Never mind that their office visit charges hover in the $50 to $60 range or higher. Never mind that their office layout, furnishings, staffing, and procedures are the same as they were eight years ago. Instead, they lash out at the messenger. Looking for someone or something to blame, even the letters to the editors of chiropractic publications seem more bitter today. The discrepancy between what is, and what should be, creates an uncomfortable feeling that is merely the first step towards an impending breakthrough.

The acceptance stage. Now, there is a calm about the doctor. Better questions are being asked. Procedures change. There is a focus and determination in rethinking the status quo that is exhilarating. While it can be painful getting to this stage, the process is essential and there are no shortcuts. With the recognition that the past isn't coming back, the doctor and staff recommit to the fundamentals of better service, increased patient education, and relevant fees. Overhead is trimmed. The status quo is questioned. Non-essentials are eliminated. Suddenly, there seems less need for the validation of expensive clothes, luxury automobiles, and private lessons. Mastering the new practice climate makes chiropractic fun again.

Some make this transition in a matter of weeks or months, and still others opt to leave the profession, because frankly, it's become too much work. This "shakeout" is separating the sheep from the goats. Those whose philosophical grounding has been limited, or who continue to depend upon third parties to define their practice, are going to feel the most disoriented. The dogma about adjusting technique, seminar leader personalities, CPT codes, practice software decisions, and the politics of the local or national association seems like so much misplaced energy.

Because it is.

Sooner or later, each practitioner will be forced to make a simple decision: am I a six-visit, symptom-relief-only chiropractor, or am I a chiropractic-lifestyle chiropractor? Pick one.

Some, still in the throes of denial will attempt to be both. "Bill, my plan is to take the six visits doled out by the managed care organization and use them to teach patients all about chiropractic and get them to continue on a cash basis after their benefits run out," they proclaim proudly.

"Let me get this straight," I respond. "You're telling me you want to join an organization that can kick you out for sneezing wrong, then let a bunch of businessmen decide what you can and can't do, and assume that it's not going to get back to headquarters that you're "brainwashing" patients into thinking the coverage they've paid for is inadequate? Is that what I hear you saying?"

"Well, yeah," they say, a little crestfallen, recognizing the folly of their optimism.

Apparently, it's as much of a stretch of the imagination for doctors to believe they can practice without depending upon third parties, as it is for patients to go from a $5 co-payment when they are sick, to feeling better and paying $35 for a non-symptomatic maintenance visit!

It's part of the eternal search for ways of having your cake and eating it too. It's a hedge. It's a game of musical chairs. It's thinking that an outsider can "time the market", buying low and selling high before the bottom falls out. It's a stalling tactic that will only serve to reduce your choices later, after the practice has lost much of its momentum. Some think that dancing with the managed care devil is merely a financial decision. It's not. It's a philosophical decision.

Chiropractors who have only heard rumors of a box on the wall from the 1960s, who have never met a chiropractor who went to jail for chiropractic, and who have been weaned on an empty calorie diet of insurance and personal injury cases, find this the hardest to accept. However, at the most fundamental level, to embrace managed care is a fear response. It's an attempt to find security. It's buying into a scarcity, zero-sum model of the world. It's a slow form of professional suicide.

"But Bill, you don't have a $20,000 monthly overhead, and live in a community where all the big employers have gone to managed care," they whimper.

"Have all the new car dealerships in your area folded? Are supermarkets just stocking beans and rice? Have all the expensive area restaurants been turned into Denny's? Are people in your community no longer shopping at the mall, going on vacation, enjoying membership at fitness clubs, or remodeling their houses?"

Perhaps the real problem is the painful realization that most people just don't value their health as much as you think they should. They'd much rather use their money to drive a late model automobile, take vacations, and eat dinners out with their families. Maybe your enemy isn't the HMO with it's shortsighted cost-containment schemes, but the fact that chiropractic has been answering a question that not enough prospective patients have been asking! After 20 years of free spinal exams, bent pens, "pain relief centers," and personal injury seminars, chiropractic has narrowed itself into a niche that is often perceived as a last resort resource for back pain or an unnecessary luxury!

Turning this around will require a long-term commitment. Dentistry is a fairly recent example of what is possible. Yes, it took 20 to 30 years to change public perceptions, and even so, millions in North Americans still don't receive any form of dental care!

Until the various chiropractic organizations can begin the grassroots educational programs necessary to equip grade school teachers with appropriate curriculum materials and classroom aids, you're stuck with patients who just don't appreciate the role of the nervous system. If you're unwilling to get in their face sufficiently to make this fundamental change, then you have built your practice and your future on unstable sand.

If you're unwilling to educate, question, probe, teach, and test your patients' understanding about chiropractic on more than just the report of findings visit, you're kissing your future goodbye. Because if you're unable to increase their perceived value of chiropractic, your only other choice is to lower your fee. If people in your community value eating dinner out with their families more than paying you for better posture, then lower your fee. If people in your community would rather drive an expensive car than have better biomechanics, then lower your fee. Just because an insurance company used to pay you $35 for an adjustment, plus another $30 for two unattended therapies, doesn't mean anyone else will. You've entered the brave new world of deregulated health care. Get used to it. ■

WHERE HAVE ALL
THE PATIENTS GONE?

Imagine picking up the latest copy of *Success Magazine* and finding classified ads selling buggy-whip franchises and ice box repair businesses! Seen any advertisements recently for replacement vacuum tubes for your radio set? When was the last time you personally changed the oil in your car? Used any coal recently? For better or worse, the world is changing. Are you keeping up? Will you be coming along with the rest of us or left behind an your indignant dogmatic rage?

FAX. 486 Computers. Windows. CD-ROM. Internet. Multimedia. Connectivity. Modems. Pixels. Cyberspace. Desktop publishing. Feeling left behind? Like the the out of touch individual who ignores a depleting bank account with the statement, "I'm not broke, I still have checks," many would just as soon stop or ignore the wheels of "progress." These modern day Amish find comfort in the golden oldies radio station, broadcasting the hits of the 1960s and 1970s. But the health care environment in which you practice is lurching into the future, with or without you.

Easy insurance money is gone. So, get over it.

Managed care, for better or worse is here. So, get used to it. The goal of a whole bunch of very smart people is to reduce your income. So, what are you going to do about it?

Suddenly, perfectly excellent chiropractors who, as students, ate a steady diet of macaroni and cheese just for the privilege of healing the sick, are questioning their career choice. The same chiropractors, who 12 years ago as students, stayed up until 3 AM debating immunization, can't make it to a two-hour meeting of local chiropractors who meet after work one Tuesday evening a month. The same fledgling chiropractors who would adjust anything that moved, just for the opportunity of being a witness to the healing process, today want to know the patient's deductible first. The same doctors who got giddy when their recommendations for 40 visits at their usual and customary fees went unquestioned, are waking up with hangovers from their third-party reimbursement party.

First, they close the door so their staff can't hear. Then, in whispered tones over the telephone they confess they're "down" by about 30% over last year. "It's the HMOs, Bill," they say in a resigned tone. "Everyone in my town is a member. The new patients have just dried up."

What they're really saying is, "Hey Bill, I just woke up from an intoxicating dream. Who's on first?" or "Gee Bill, it looks like I'm not competitive anymore." Or more simply, "I'm scared."

If they don't blame the local HMO, they blame the insurance-numbed patient. "They're just not used to paying for health care out of their own pockets," they grouse.

True, clearly stating a problem is the first step towards solving it. But these doctors are in the I-can't-believe-it stage of realization. Now, they wish they'd educated their patients. Now, they wish they'd conducted regular progress examinations and reports. Now, they wish they'd gotten out of debt. Now, they wish they'd stayed in touch with all their past patients. Now, they wish they hadn't been so fixated on getting new patients. Now, they wish they hadn't made their patients angry with annoying recall scripts. Now, they wish they'd done things differently.

When you're through grieving over what you should've, could've, would've done, pick a few of these action steps and get to work!

1. Adopt an abundance mentality. Remember the argument for having the government swallow up 1/7th of the GNP and socialize health care? Estimates suggested that 37 million people weren't covered by any kind of formal health care plan. The members of this group in your community have no allegiance to any HMO, independent medical examiner, or capitation plan. They drive past your clinic every day. In fact, listen carefully enough and you can hear them right now! No new patients? Really?

If HMOs and managed care are such bad things, which chiropractor in your community is going after the resulting disenfranchised, frustrated, and compromised patient? Putting health care under the control of bean-counting bureaucrats didn't make medicine suddenly more effective! Who's asking for the patients who have been told "to learn to live with it" or that "it's all in your head"? Who's putting out the welcome mat for patients whose problems have been minimized, ignored, or asked to wait for days and days or hours and hours to see a doctor for three minutes?

Action step: Recognize that there are plenty of patients "out there." Why aren't your current patients referring others? What could you do to make it easier for them to do so? Have you asked them? Can patients "smell" the fear on you? Can patients tell you're not having fun? Why would they want to refer a friend to a doctor who lacks confidence or seems preoccupied and distracted? It may win you an Oscar nomination, but you'd better get that chin up and at least start pretending to have fun. No one wants to consult a loser.

2. Work on your trophy case. For years this profession has been consumed with getting new patients. And, for years new patients have been treated like one-night stands by macho doctors looking to "prove" that chiropractic works to one more skeptical, last-resort-insurance-policy-toting patient. Once symptomatic results were obtained, few patients were incentivized to continue with wellness care. Instead, as they were starting to feel better, they had to cool their heels in the reception room, waiting for the next crop of time-consuming symptomatic patients to go through their exams and reports. Then, they were asked to pay full retail for a non-symptomatic "tune-up." While they weren't formally asked to leave, they felt increasingly uncomfortable or unwelcome in an environment that seemed singularly designed for fawning over a constant parade of hurting patients.

Sitting on your shelf are countless patient files. These are special people who braved conventional wisdom and ventured into your office. What they probably found was a likable doctor. They probably got great results. And could vouch for you to others that chiropractic is a valid discipline worth investigating. But no, you were more interested in the next new patient, a new conquest!

Action step: Like the one night stand, you didn't call. You didn't stay in touch. In fact, you're a little embarrassed that you weren't more civilized. So, apologize. Sure. Send inactive patients a letter apologizing for not keeping in touch and offer them an incentive (a free reactivation visit?) to rekindle the relationship. Chances are, most of your patients would find the humility of your outreach quite attractive, giving you a chance to re-establish contact and see what's new at your office. Would your office be in such a sorry state if just 10% of all the patients you'd ever seen, started coming in just once a month? Who needs more new patients when you've already seen enough new patients to last a lifetime?

3. Install an appropriate fee system. Your customer has changed. It used to be that insurance companies were your customers. They had deep pockets and could justify lots of diagnostics and a fee structure. Now your customer is increasingly a cash patient who must accommodate your fees within an already burdened personal budget. To add insult to injury, for some, your fees may be on top of the contribution they've already made to their ineffective HMO!

Ever hear the stories about the five dollar adjustments back in late 1960s and early 1970s before insurance "equality?" True, that's when you could buy a postage stamp for a nickel and a loaf of bread for a quarter. I'm no economist, but it seems to me that the usual and customary charges in offices today, have ballooned much larger than the cost of living in the last 30 years. What would the cost of an adjustment be today if the insurance era had never happened?

The problem of course, is that many doctors unwisely based their ability to pay 30 year mortgages on the incomes provided by insurance company policies. And tightening the belt doesn't feel, well, doctorly. Lowering fees doesn't seem successful. Reducing your staff isn't pleasant. There are worse things than recognizing you misjudged the future!

Action step: Give your financial policy a good looking over. True, patients can afford anything they want, but when they want that new car, new boat, or dream vacation, it is almost always paid on credit. And while you didn't go to chiropractic college to become a banker, your ability to offer affordable fees, a variety of ways patients can pay for their care (case fee, fee for service, barter, etc.), and frankly your ability to carry patient receivables over a period of time, may be critical aspects of how well you adapt.

Change is never easy. The choices may seem hopelessly out of step with what you're accustomed to, but 1985 isn't coming back! ■

EMPTY CALORIES

It has almost become a cliche that if something tastes good, it probably isn't good for you. The reverse seems true as well. Exercise, whole grain foods, and shunning refined sugar requires continuous discipline and a desensitization process to adapt to the subtle flavors and long-term benefits. The allure of the sweetness, the satisfaction from the fat content, and the silky textures of packaged foods are difficult to overcome. But then, so is the temptation to join every HMO around.

Like the empty calories of junk food and the lack of nutrition and "staying power" that more wholesome foods contain, many chiropractic doctors aren't reading the nutrition labels on their HMO contracts. The mythology that surrounds this subject is causing many doctors to make poor decisions.

Myth #1 Everybody's doing it. Remember when you wanted to do something dumb, your mom or dad would ask, "If your friends wanted you to jump off a cliff, would you do that, too?" Same thing here. Just because other chiropractors are signing away their ability to control their destinies, doesn't mean you should. Remember, when a whole bunch of people believe in a bad idea, it's still a bad idea. A better question is why does this "lemming" outlook seem so attractive to a profession of iconoclastic Lone Rangers? Is wanting to be included and accepted that strong? Is the inability to communicate the value of chiropractic that prevalent?

Myth #2 I might miss something. Of course, one of the fear tactics used to snare chiropractors to participate is that the whole health care industry is going to cost containment and managed care, and if you don't participate, you'll be left out in the cold without any patients. If your new patient statistics are down (and for many they are) and you yearn for the magic days of plentiful insurance, you might actually believe this notion. However, getting on the list, having your treatment plans questioned by bureaucrats who don't understand what you do, and then having your fee basis slowly cut until you're actually losing money to see an HMO patient, is something you might want to pass up. If you're losing money on every patient, you can't make it up with volume. How much does it cost you to render a chiropractic adjustment? (Total monthly overhead divided by the number of monthly paid visits.)

Myth #3 I'll automatically get patients. One reason why doctors are submitting to the uncomfortable bit in their mouths and the controlling harnesses offered by managed care, is because indemnity insurance has practically disappeared. That, combined with the perception that more and more patients are being "covered" by an HMO, causes many doctors to wave a white flag and surrender. The promise that they'll get an endless stream of new patients without lifting a marketing finger is quickly confirmed as merely part of the sales pitch. (Many HMOs just want to claim that they have chiropractors on board.) Few chiropractors enjoy the new patient volumes stated in the sales presentation.

Worse than the dribble of new patients is the mountains of paperwork and approvals needed to render chiropractic care. Subscribing chiropractors quickly ascertain that they've traded their freedom for even more paperwork, more stress, more unappreciative patients who expect miracles in six visits or less, and someone watching their every move.

Myth #4 It's just a new form of insurance. Painting managed care as just a derivative of insurance is like suggesting rap music is kind of like the music that accompanies a square dance call! Yes, both types of music feature a sing-song speaking pattern, but they are clearly two different genres! Same with major medical insurance and managed care. It's the next thing, but that doesn't make it good.

72

Making money-grubbing doctors the enemy is counterproductive, nor does it address the true cause of the health care "crisis." But like other forms of symptom treating, it offers short term gratification and side steps the discipline and the public education required to make true progress.

Myth #5 HMOs love chiropractic. Most managed care organizations don't understand chiropractic and barely find it acceptable treatment for the symptomatic treatment of low back pain! The attitudes and entrenchment of the traditional mechanistic model of physiology are so prevalent, chiropractic is a nuisance. When one HMO in Texas picked their participating chiropractors by holding a lottery, you know that standards of care, experience, and accessibility aren't the governing criteria! They simply want the right to advertise that they have chiropractors in their network. How does it feel to be the token chiropractor? Affirmative action meets health care.

Myth #6 I'll help reduce costs and "prove" chiropractic. This is an enviable goal, but your experience is likely to degenerate into the newly commissioned 24-year old stockbroker thinking some 65-year old millionaire is going to take him seriously. An HMO is a business, not a research laboratory. Taking risks and trying new things is not the motive. There may be rare exceptions, however managed care organizations are about one thing; turning a profit. Instead of listening to your impassioned plea for cost/benefit studies, it's just easier to cut your reimbursement or reduce the number of times you're allowed to see the patient. This is symptom treating at its very best. "Don't confuse me with the facts, I've already made up my mind."

Myth #7 I won't be able to survive without joining. Now, we're getting somewhere. You may have it backwards. If you join, and your income is slowly cut back, and you become further distracted by the non-clinical aspects of membership, and you finally cry "Uncle," you'll have lost even more momentum than the decline of major medical insurance has caused. When you are dismissed in favor of a bright-eyed and bushy-tailed new graduate who will work for even less, you'll wonder why you took this little detour in the first place. Chiropractic is bigger than any managed care scheme.

Myth #8 Patients won't pay for chiropractic out of their own pockets. Boy, does this show one's true colors! Certainly there are countless patients who, as you read this, are submitting to back surgery because it's covered by their HMO. It's a big leap from there, to the notion patients won't pay for care. How were chiropractors compensated before insurance equality and third party "acceptance?" "Yeah, but they were only making five dollars an adjustment," you correctly observe. True. Figure out what inflation and the cost of living increases have done to that five dollar office visit. I bet it didn't increase to the $35 or $50 some chiropractors expect their cash paying patients to pay! (Just because your 30 year home mortgage was based upon $100 deductibles, doesn't mean patients will pay the fees you charged back in 1986!)

Myth #9 I'll convert them to wellness patients. This is the secret strategy of many chiropractors who have accepted the straitjacket of managed care. While this is probably the healthiest response, it is a course fraught with dangerous reefs and unpredictable currents. Since most managed care organizations can dismiss you for parting your hair on the wrong side, or just about any other clinical or nonclinical reason, be careful! Once word gets back to headquarters from patients who are indignant that their policy doesn't cover "adequate" chiro-practic care (as defined by you), instead of getting to explain the research, or the literature, or justifying your patient indoctrination program, you'll merely get a pink slip. The same day, another chiropractor miraculously gets "accepted" into the program. It's not nice to fool Mother HMO.

Myth #10 The future is hopeless. This is an exciting time for chiropractic. The public is increasingly fed up with the medical model, the knee-jerk prescriptions, and the holier-than-thou attitude. Research shows that in growing numbers, people are consulting non-mainstream health care providers. In Australia, where chiroprac-tic is excluded in the national health plan, and spinal manipulation is available at virtually no cost from medical practitioners, chiropractic is thriving. In British Columbia, where the provincial government pays for 12 visits and no X-rays, the chiropractors who opt out of the system seem to be having the most fun. True, it requires the ability to deliver the goods, educate patients, and communicate the value of chiropractic, but that's what makes chiropractic fun. If patient education, rapport, and persuasive communications aren't your cup of tea, or, you've reduced chiropractic to merely a non-invasive form of therapy for headaches and low back pain, then managed care might seem pretty attractive.

Managed health care isn't about health or caring. It's about management. If it seems enticing, or you're tempted by the packaging and window dressing, realize the implications of your decision. Because, it requires the fundamental mistrust of the homeostatic relationship between doctor and patient to make third party involvement palatable. Accepting a third party policeman into the relationship to skim the profits due you by your training, your sacrifice, and your commitment to the truth, is perhaps one of the most sublime examples of practice sabotage and professional suicide. ■

COMMITTING SUICIDE

As the worst fears of more and more doctors come true and they see their practices slowly erode, many contemplate ways to make up the difference in their declining incomes. The desperateness of these schemes and the counterproductive results that accrue are sad testimonials to the chiropractic philosophy of cause and effect. Deluded into treating symptoms, countless doctors are abandoning one of the most powerful ideas in the world to chase after illusions, shadows, and the hope of making the money they used to make, or feel they deserve to make.

If you can't figure out how to adapt to today's changing practice climate, the following may give you some ideas.

1. Multi-level marketing. This seems so attractive. With all the people you see, you should be able to make a killing with vitamins, enzyme supplements, or water purifiers! Sure, take your eye off chiropractic and get excited about something new. Since people apparently don't want chiropractic, create a "down line" that can produce income while you sleep. If you'd put this much focus on your practice, you wouldn't be interested in "going Diamond."

2. HMO membership. The fear tactics used to entrap doctors into these arrangements should be your first clue! Thinking that an organization committed to reducing health care costs is going to gratefully fulfill your marketing needs by supplying an endless stream of new patients is a pipe dream. Do you believe in the Tooth Fairy and Santa Claus, too?

3. Get another degree. Maybe the reason you're not making enough money is that you don't know enough. Chances are you have the book knowledge of chiropractic well under control. Certainly, escaping into the protective cove of a school or a series of twelve consecutive seminars can buy you some time, but that's not the problem. Adding more initials after your name is unlikely to improve the fundamentals of your patient relationships.

4. Move your practice. Here's a popular idea. Seems the grass is always greener somewhere else. Maybe you want to live where it's not so cold. Maybe you want to get closer to your aging parents. Or, maybe you want to find someplace where the insurance money is still good. Starting over someplace new and forcing yourself to get excited about practice again (because you have to), is an interesting (and wasteful) strategy.

5. Open another office. After living in the area for awhile you notice that just 16 miles away there's an area that doesn't have the usual wall-to-wall carpet coverage of chiropractors. The notion of opening a satellite clinic enters your mind and just won't go away. Welcome to an interesting phenomenon called $1 + 1 = 1$. If you thought running the office you practice in is challenging, just wait until you have to motivate someone else in a remote office to help slay the overhead dragon. Or would you rather divide your time between both offices. Enjoy the commute!

6. Hire an associate. Here the thinking must be that someone sharp enough whom you'd trust with your patients and your practice, will allow him or herself to be exploited for slave wages. Even if you can find someone, it's ironic that expanding your office hours rarely compensates for the headaches, lack of focus, and ego encounters you're likely to endure. Do you really like managing others, or do you just need the distraction of finding out the hard way?

7. Add rehab. Maybe you're just not providing enough services. Could it be that going into debt to add the machines, computers, staff, and additional overhead is just a way to light a fire under yourself? Oh sure, it's easy to rationalize the patient benefits of chiropractic combined with state-of-the-art muscle and soft tissue rehabilitation, but could your interest be prompted by the good insurance reimbursement these non-chiropractic services still enjoy?

8. Seek hospital privileges. For doctors who need to be reminded of their victim status to get fired up about chiropractic, this one is a natural. Now you can devote countless hours of meetings and political, behind-the-scenes maneuvering to bring chiropractic to the increasingly empty beds at the local hospital. The obstacles to overcome and the injustice of being excluded simply stokes the fire.

9. Start a seminar. Now, this is a wonderful distraction. Things are working so well at your office, you'll want to spread the good cheer to other unsuspecting chiropractors! Learn all about working with the sales and catering departments of hotels. Argue with your graphic designer about your seminar mailer advertising. Spend thousands of dollars on promotion and enjoy the glamour of airports, the stunning company of hotel bellmen, and the surprises of meeting room AV technicians. Better yet, you'll get to spend even more time away from your demanding family. Perfect!

10. Second-guess the successful. Maybe you're just too good to be saddled with an actual practice. Have you considered a career as an independent medical examiner? The pay is good and you get to superimpose your narrow vision of chiropractic on those unethical doctors treating families (even children!) for more than the allotted eight visits for low back pain. Just think, a steady supply of patients and regular checks from a thankful insurance company. Just like the old days.

11. Join a practice management firm. While less of a commitment than getting another degree, making it to the monthly seminars is, well, almost fun. Maybe there are some CPT codes you've overlooked. Maybe there are some special words or incantations you can utter while in front of the X-ray view box that will compel patients to do your bidding. Maybe. But don't hold your breath. You didn't even follow all the recommendations from the last practice management program you attended. And, that cost $6,000.

12. Sell your practice to an unsuspecting student. If all else fails, find a student with deep-pocket relatives and sell your practice while there's still time! Never mind that those file folders of inactive patients you've put such a high value on will never return. Never mind that the student is likely to default on his note. Never mind. Because you're history.

The allure of many of these ideas is that it feels like you're actually doing something proactive to improve your circumstances. Many of these tactics make it seem like you're moving forward, expanding, improving, offering new services, and generally evolving your practice or increasing your chiropractic commitment. Yet, the sad truth is that they are all examples of selfish egotism that simply distract you from getting your hands dirty by actually serving patients. Deeply serving patients. Passionately serving patients. Uninhibitedly serving patients.

Have you ever heard that if you want to get something done, give it to someone busy? That's because there's always a job for a servant. A true servant. Those who want to practice by remote control or who can only produce value for patients when a third party pays for it, need new careers. Missiles, mortershells, and high altitude bombing won't do. Guerrilla warfare is required. Hand-to-hand combat skills are essential. If you hesitate, if you're unsure, if you reveal your uncertainty or disorientation, you're dead. Some will self-inflict their wounds so they can retire from the front lines. Others will commit professional suicide by devoting their energies to other off-purpose pursuits. Meanwhile, those rare individuals who truly own chiropractic will be insanely busy healing a hurting world. ∎

FAIR WEATHER PHILOSOPHY

A common cry among chiropractors these days is that more and more patients are revealing that they don't want chiropractic "because my HMO doesn't pay for it." This has caused even the most confident clinicians to succumb to panic, fear, and ultimately anger. Enough incidents like this in a slower-than-normal month can prompt even the most rational chiropractors to rethink the value of their freedom and contemplate the safety and security of joining every HMO or PPO program possible. As patients increasingly become pawns in the money-making schemes of the medical-industrial complex, chiropractors often see themselves as helpless victims.

Not even in the days when some chiropractors found themselves going to jail, has there been so much fear and disillusionment. It is little help that chiropractors are willing to admit that they squandered valuable opportunities to adequately educate millions of patients who showed up with $100 deductibles. "What can I do right now to get things turned around," plead chiropractors as their voices become more shrill.

Here are ten things you could start doing this very minute. You won't have to buy anything, take your staff to a seminar, or sign up for a one year contract. Of course, like chiropractic itself, these suggestions may be too simple, too obvious, or decline to give you the instant gratification you'd like. But here they are anyway.

1. Cut overhead. What could be more obvious? Rethink virtually every practice expense. Ask yourself how each expenditure will either increase patient understanding, improve productivity, or pro-vide a service your patients want and are willing to pay for.

2. Reduce entanglements. Get out of unproductive associate relationships. Fire the staff that are not pulling their weight. Stop taking insurance assignment. Simplify!

3. Refocus your purpose. Get reacquainted with your purpose and why you chose chiropractic. What's standing in the way of your destiny? What fear or artificial barrier is blinding you to living your dream? Find it. And ruthlessly pierce through its bondage over you by facing it squarely without blinking. Write it down. Focus!

4. Educate like crazy. Make sure your patients understand what you do, why you do it, and are able to defend their chiropractic decision to anyone they encounter. Use each office visit to pop a question that a friend or family member might ask them, and allow your patients to rehearse their answer in the safety of your office.

5. Adjust your personal overhead. Virtually every financial issue raised by a doctor is a spending problem, not an earning problem. If your personal lifestyle is still based upon your 1987 income, wake up. It may not be pretty, but you're going to have to break it to your spouse that times have changed. Even if your income has been cut by 30% or more, you're still probably making more money than most of your patients.

6. Increase patient volume. Today, more than ever, creating the accessibility, implementing the office procedures, and removing the capacity blockages that limit patient volumes during the busiest times of the day are essential. Make it easier for patients to get what they want from you—when they want it.

7. Lower your fees. Since you don't have to give up dinner out with your family or make other sacrifices with your disposable income to get an adjustment, this may be the hardest to swallow. The fact is, very few doctors have the personality, the tableside manners, the patient education, or the compelling office protocols that would make patients feel an adjustment is worth $35. That was the fee for insurance companies, remember? But insurance companies are less and less an issue these days!

8. Increase patient feedback. Many doctors are still inclined to deliver the same tired report of findings or lay lecture that worked in 1987. Instead of performing a "data dump", ask more questions. Understand your patients better. Find out what they think. Make your chiropractic explanations more relevant.

9. Become more outspoken. This is not the time to cower in the corner! Take the initiative. Take a stand. Return to the conservative, inside-out, philosophy that the world is asking for. Be a crusader for self-responsibility. Be a vocal opponent to intervention by big government, big insurance companies, or big anything. Become a passionate advocate for the truth. Make waves. Get in people's faces.

10. Become a better servant. This may be the most important of all. You've chosen a life of professional service. How come you're so worried about yourself and your own needs? How come you're more concerned about your plummeting income instead of the needless surgeries foisted upon innocent patients? Find better ways to serve. Your patients are suffering more than you are! Eternal job security is guaranteed to those who will truly serve.

Interestingly, when these simple, practical and rational suggestions are offered, many chiropractors choose to ignore or deny them. Hope springs eternal, so these doctors go from one seminar to the next, and call one practice "expert" after another. Most seem to be looking for some inexpensive gimmick or script or "thing" that can produce enough increased patient flow to reassure themselves that chiropractic still works and that the future is going to be all right.

As more and more time is wasted catering to these denial strategies, each doctor's resources and momentum dwindles. Desperately grasping at even the smallest shred of floating debris from the sinking shipwreck of the insurance era, chiropractors seem prepared to sell out their philosophy, their uniqueness, and a 100 year history of drugless healing. If your philosophy of treating "cause" works for patients, why not apply it to your own practice?

The notion that patients can't seem to afford chiropractic is a symptom. The idea that patients prefer surgery because it will be paid for by a third party is a symptom. The reality that patients drop out of care once they feel better is a symptom. The fact that your patient financial policy is no longer relevant to today's practice climate is a symptom. The observation that the yellow page ads and free spinal exams of the past no longer work is a symptom.

I thought you preferred to be the doctor of cause.

Do you have the courage, self-confidence, and focus to confront the real cause of the challenges facing you and your practice? Or, will you be unable to rise above the compelling siren's song offering "security" by being a whipping boy of some unappreciative managed care organization?

Deny it if you wish. Ignore it if you want. Overlook it if you must. But here's the truth: Your patients and your community are crying for leadership. Everyone is waiting for you to stand up for the truth. We are tired of political correctness and are waiting for someone to declare the truth. Do you have it in you?

Or do you choose the path of least resistance? True, it is wide, well traveled, and flat. Yes, it's more crowded than the more difficult trail. Sure, the signs are easy to read and there are even guard rails at every curve. But the smooth ride afforded here dulls the senses and tames the soul. The destination is just a mirage, constantly advancing in the shimmering future. Instead of the satisfaction afforded those who overcome great odds and advance the truth, the reward is a shallow mediocrity that insults the spirit.

It's your decision. ∎

LIVING OFF TABLE SCRAPS

For native American Indians living on the plains, the buffalo hunt was one of the most important sources of food. Slaying these huge animals was done in a most creative manner. When a herd was spotted, lazily grazing away, scouting parties would surround the herd and create a stampede, causing numbers of buffalo to be herded over cliffs and plummet to their deaths. A similar technique is being used on chiropractors!

As the last drops of insurance money are sucked from the nipples of third parties, more and more doctors are turning to managed care, in a furtive attempt to maintain their $100 deductible lifestyles of the 1980s. Fooled into thinking that HMOs and PPOs and IPAs and all the other acronyms, are merely a contemporary rendition of the juicy insurance policies of the 1980s, countless chiropractors are extending their tin plates, hoping to be included in the latest scheme to disburse health care dollars.

Unlike the indemnity policies of the past, managed care organizations are about management, not care. In fact, so good at management are these organizations, a recent *Wall Street Journal* article indicated they have collectively stashed away over $9 billion dollars in the bank! In the process of raiding the health care industry they have reduced doctors to "providers" and picked off the weakest by tempting them with the false validation of being included. Thousands of doctors (in all disciplines) are waking up to find that their years of schooling, countless hours of continuing education, and the risk of running a small business have been reduced to a job. Sneeze wrong, refuse to go along, tell a patient they need more care than mandated by their HMO, and you're out.

Threatened that you couldn't survive outside the system, doctors who have watched their practices slowly erode are hoping to be one of the "chosen." As the cliff looms closer and closer, and doctors are finding their professional lives flashing before them, they can find solace in the fact that patients are suffering from this new arrangement even more than doctors.

Oh yes, there are a few isolated cases where doctors and patients are living in a new utopian bliss, orchestrated by a bunch of bureaucrats second-guessing doctor's recommendations from their cubicles bathed in fluorescent light, but they are few and far between. Remember, the sole motive of managed care is to increase premiums as much as the market will bear, and reduce payments to you until your resources are so diminished you must get a second job to make ends meet, or you cry "Uncle!" and bolt for the door. Unfortunately, many doctors are choosing the former, looking over multi-level opportunities with new interest.

The solutions to this new challenge aren't pretty. In fact, they may be so distasteful that instead, many will hope to survive the fall to the bottom of the ravine by breaking their fall on the bodies of doctors already there. Don't count on it.

If you're already entangled in managed care or contemplating taking the plunge, here are some things to consider:

1. Managed care is built on a false idea. Even with all the talk about preventive care hidden in the fine print, managed care is about treating symptoms. Actually, treating symptoms in the fastest, cheapest way and with little concern about the future or the likelihood of relapse. Gone are the archaic monikers of "straight" or "mixer." Now the issue is, are you a symptom-treater of neuromuscular skeletal conditions in six visits or less, or are you a chiropractic lifestyle chiropractor? Trying to wear both hats, trying to serve two masters, will be met with frustration that will lead many to question their career choice.

Yes, managed care is one of those issues that will force chiropractors to revisit their philosophy and make the hard choice of shunning managed care, or selling out to chase the table scraps that will hopefully cover the Lexus payments.

If you can live with the ambiguity and feel that you must embrace managed care, make sure that income from this source is no more than 25% of your gross income. Make sure it cannot overwhelm you. Make sure it remains a small fish in your big pond of other types of patients.

2. Managed care will force changes in financial policy. As the ebb and flow of circumstances change, the "going rate" for the benchmark of care (the chiropractic adjustment) will change too. Offices will either be forced to work even harder to increase a patient's perceived value of care, leaving their current financial policy in place, or succumb to market pressures and lower their fees. There are only two choices.

If your fee structure is still lingering at the high tide watermark of the insurance era so PI lawyers find your office hospitable, you'll be in for the rudest awakening. As your books get cluttered with all kinds of creative "Individual Consideration Contracts" and financial hardship arrangements that sabotage the efforts of your staff to collect at the front desk, practice will become increasingly stressful. All this, while HMO patients shun your office because you're not a subscriber to their plan, or patients no longer respect you because they think you're only worth their $8 co-payment. Sounds like fun!

The hard truth is that you must be prepared to pour increasingly high levels of energy into your patient education efforts, or you must lower your fees. Dream if you wish, but 1986 isn't coming back! Be prepared to work harder and make less money—see more people at a lower fee. Fact is, what you're charging your financial hardship cases *is* your usual and customary fee! The rare personal injury case and major medical patient are merely statistical anomalies!

3. Rethink your personal and professional overhead. Why did you get involved in chiropractic? I bet it was to help people, defend the truth, offer alternatives to useless drugs and irreversible surgery. I bet it had little to do with making a lot of money, driving a fancy car, and being thought of as a big shot. However, it's the car payments, house payments, lessons for the kids, club memberships, and other amenities that are blinding you to the changing practice environment around you. Selling the car or giving up the club membership is, well, you know, embarrassing.

Swallow your pride and get real! Lifestyle decisions based on a 1986 insurance-based practice with tasty personal injury cases are no longer relevant. Rethink your practice, your procedures, and ways you can reduce your personal financial obligations. Batten down the hatches. Make your practice shipshape. Tighten your belt. It's going to get worse, perhaps much worse, before it gets better. The bottom line is, the market will no longer bear the frills or the extravagance of the past.

4. Develop your interpersonal communication skills. Time was you could get a license, buy a computer, hire some "girls," place a yellow page ad, and take a few lawyers out to lunch and you could build an enviable source of income. Not today.

Now, instead of lining up patients ten deep and face down on unattended therapy, each with insurance policies hanging out of their pockets, practice today requires new combat skills. No longer can you afford to remain a technique nerd with the bashful personality of a pimply-faced teenager. You must be passionate, communicative, and your tableside manners must be confident and nurturing. You must have a personality. If you don't have one, get one!

Now, you must be able to confront a patient face to face. Hand-to-hand combat requires different tools, a different sense of timing, and a different set of personal skills that, for many doctors, atrophied or never developed during the 1980s. Get to a Toastmasters group and practice your ability to arrange your ideas into understandable concepts. Read books on customer service that have nothing to do with chiropractic. Recognize that this is a time of tremendous change and opportunity. Ignore it like Rip Van Winkle and the world will pass you by. ∎

COMPETING AGAINST MANAGED CARE

A story passed around the advertising industry is about a brewery in Wisconsin that watched its market share steadily decrease until to the point of almost bankruptcy. The brewer hired a famous advertising agency to help turn around the sales decline. The agency people studied the brewery facility from top to bottom. They asked questions. They analyzed the advertising of the competition. The recommendation? Advertise the fact that they used a particular type of hops in the production of their beer. "But every brewery uses the same type of hops," argued the brewery president in dismay. "True, but no other brewery has turned it into a unique quality," came the reply. History records a major turnaround for the brewer. As managed care providers pummel those chiropractors who are not members, a similar opportunity presents itself.

A week doesn't pass that I don't get calls from doctors challenged by patients who tell their doctor in effect, "You're not on my list, I can't see you any more." The script may vary slightly, but the result is that the patient is looking at the bottom line cost as a basis for making their health care decisions. (This problem isn't new. Chiropractors have long complained about patients who needlessly submit to surgical intervention because "it's covered by my insurance.") And while this may be hard to understand for someone who values their health as much as you do, finances play a role for patients who must actually pay for their care.

Having patients seduced by the low cost provider is the same problem that countless mom and pop retail stores have faced as the new Wal-Mart comes to town and opens its doors. Sadly, many small businesses succumbed to the path of least resistance, closing their doors after years of service to their communities. More and more chiropractors are facing a similar choice. Stay and fight, or make that video rental store a dream come true.

Maybe you didn't get in to the local network. Maybe you didn't want in. However, combating the chiropractic offices that *did* join requires a similar approach as used by the brewery and the small businesses thriving in the shadow of huge retailing behemoths. It is not business as usual. Roll up your sleeves, put on your marketing hat, and let the games begin!

First, recognize that one of your most valuable assets are your inactive patient files—people who know you, know where your office is, know your wonderful tableside manners, and know of the great results you produce. If you haven't been nurturing these patients through letters, postcards, newsletters, occasional patient appreciation days, annual check up offers, and the like, get started! Out of all the people on the planet, these are the people most likely to make an appearance in your office. It can seem like a long, one-sided conversation, but persevere. There are no better prospects. Even if you're new in practice and only have 20 inactive files, keep in touch with these patients. Forever! Think of their care as simply in the dormant stage. Keep the relationship going. Make sure every one of those patients would feel that they'd be welcomed back without an "I told you so" and be delighted to encounter you while shopping for groceries. Think long term.

Second, carefully analyze your competition. A famous marketing axiom suggests: "1. Price, 2. Speed, 3. Quality. Pick any two." This rule of thumb is helpful in uncovering the Achilles heel of any competitor. If your competitor is selling on price (such as managed care seems to be doing), then they almost always have to concede speed or quality. Whatever factor they seem to be neglecting should become a major focus of your marketing efforts. This is how small businesses have been successful in co-existing beside large retailers who can offer the lowest prices.

Third, in light of the rule of thumb above, it's time you grab a yellow pad of paper and begin taking an inventory of the unique factors of your practice. Most businesses do this as a matter of course when designing a marketing plan. You've never had one. So, let's get started. Here are some ideas and strategic observations that may help get you started:

1. Practice resources. Do you have special equipment, tools, procedures, that you can claim as yours by being the first to make them an issue? Do you take for granted what your flexion/distraction table offers your patients? Have you become numb to the patient convenience of your hi-lo table? Have you overlooked the convenience of your in-house massage therapist? Your X-ray equipment?

2. Your devotion to the patient's health. If you've decided to go solo, without some profit-motivated bureaucracy looking over your shoulder to second-guess your recommendations, you can be totally focused on the patient's health. "Our patient's don't have their problem minimized so as to fit some statistical model. We take your health seriously! It is our only concern." Your objectivity can be positioned as a patient benefit.

3. Years of experience. If you've been doing this more than ten years or so, your experience "with a wide variety of cases" can be perceived as a competitive advantage. How many patients have you helped? How many hours of post-graduate continuing education have you received? What special degrees, certification, or training have you acquired?

4. Same day appointments. Do you have openings each day for new patients? Without specifically mentioning this it is easy for a first time chiropractic patient to think they'll have to wait until next week, like getting into their medical doctor's office. If you offer same day appointments it is a marketable service.

5. Number of successful cases helped. How many headache patients have you helped? What's your success rate? If you've never thought about it or kept track, get busy! What better way to bolster a patient's confidence and create a competitive advantage than to identify your batting average? To differentiate managed-care chiropractic from patient-directed chiropractic care, you have to roll up your sleeves.

6. Patient conveniences. It may not seem relevant to where you practice, but what about parking? Is it easy? Is it free? Is there easy access for traffic in either directions in front of your office? What about office hours? Are you practicing the same hours as the managed care facility down the street? Why? Maybe it's time to reclaim Thursdays and make it your big day. How about at least one Saturday a month? Rethink the status quo.

7. Affordable care. If you want to go head-to-head, lower your overhead, cinch up your belt, and make your fee structure competitive. If you wish you were a member of a network and were excluded, why not offer care for the same cut rate fee you would have been offering as a member, sans paperwork, hassle, and second-guessing? Price should be the last thing you negotiate, but if that's the writing on the wall you're reading, then what are your other choices?

8. Patient education. Believe it or not, the very mention of the fact that you "explain everything in advance" can be a significant competitive advantage. Like many of the other points mentioned, you probably take your patient education efforts for granted. What makes your patient education uniquely beneficial to today's time-conscious patient?

9. Community involvements. Don't laugh. You'd be surprised how many fellow Rotarians, Red Cross volunteers, or Annual Pooh-Bah fund raiser contributors will seek out one of their own. Keep your community involvements to yourself and you overlook an aspect which could give others a reason for choosing your office over the next.

10. Your staff accomplishments. I bet your staff has some special training or particular skills that make your office compelling to prospective new patients. Is it a great personality, skilled with children, helpful over the phone, able to get answers, sensitivity to the needs of new patients, or professional nursing experience?

11. Doctor access. Are you accessible by telephone to answer questions? That's a competitive advantage that a lot of patients would find appealing. Your willingness to field questions, clear up concerns, and discuss issues without forcing the patient to make a seemingly irreversible commitment to show up in your office could pay huge dividends. Already do it? Well how come your current patients don't know this so they can urge their friends to call?

12. Patient testimonials. Forget the dog-eared book in the reception room—by the time those testimonials are read you're preaching to the choir! Do you have patients who would be willing to field an occasional phone call from a prospective patient who is considering care in your office? An office so open and confident, with patients willing to vouch for them, could be turned into a competitive advantage.

13. Thorough examination. Again, you probably figure every chiropractor delivers a thorough examination so it's not differentiating factor. Perhaps you need to make it a factor! How many different tests do you typically conduct? How good are you at detecting other problems that patients forget to mention? How many times have you uncovered problems that prompted you to refer out? "Does your managed care provider deliver a thorough examination, or are you rushed through like a number?"

As you can see there are many aspects of your practice that you take for granted that can be turned into irresistible reasons to consult your office. Once you assemble your list, make sure your active and inactive patients know this information about your office! Some of these items probably belong in your yellow page ad. Print the most important ones on the back of your business card. Act! You're playing catch up ball now, and every day counts. ■

JOINING UP

As managed care and tightening economic times continue to take a bite out of an increasing number of doctor's incomes, more and more are investigating management firms. Thinking that there must be someone, somewhere with a "secret to success", many are inclined to sign up with a practice management consultant. I frequently field phone calls from doctors on the verge of taking this big step and are having some last-minute jitters. It's probably this inability to make decisions that has prompted them to consider handing over $600 a month. Never mind. In our consumer-oriented culture, we're used to solving our problems by buying something.

I try to listen courteously to the gnashing of teeth, or the victim mentality, or the scarcity outlook, or the notion that their community has a unique medical orientation, or the grousing about the new doctors down the block "giving away everything," or the hundred and one other excuses for their current predicament. After about five minutes or so I ask the calling doctor, "What measurable outcome do you hope to achieve from joining a management firm?"

Suddenly, the most emotional and intuitive doctors become incredibly analytical! In an attempt to justify the emotional strings pulled by the management firm at its introductory teaser seminar, the callers generally explain a lack of patient volume, a desire for more free time, or quote some arbitrary statistical model they think they should be living up to. I can tell that these doctors have already made up their minds to join, but I humor them, and continue.

"The way I see it, there are only about five reasons to join a management firm," I observe.

"Really? What are they?" they ask, apparently thinking that what they need for practice success is going to come from the outside in.

1. Belong to something big. Many doctors have heard stories of big chiropractic pep rallies at the Hyatt Hotel and they want to belong. Isolated in their practices, abused by an unappreciative staff, beaten up by insurance company IMEs, ignored by patients, and hounded by a spouse accustomed to an ever increasingly higher standard of living, many doctors hope membership in a chiropractic "country club" will offer security and a sympathetic ear. Whether it's Joe Sixpack commiserating down at Joe's Bar over a beer, or doctors talking in hushed tones in the hallways at the Hyatt, misery loves company. Joining a management firm allows the doctor to lick his or her wounds in the company of others who need a shoulder to cry on. No wonder patients don't refer or follow recommendations.

2. Buy some discipline. In this scenario, the doctor recognizes he or she lacks the personal discipline to do what's best for the practice. It may be a lack of confrontation skills. It may be an ineffective report of findings. Or, the lack of systems to assure a consistent protocol. Apparently, these doctors need the weekly telephone badgering of a consultant to follow through with the more distasteful aspects of practice. Never mind that the consultant has never actually been in the office environment in which the doctor practices. Never mind that they've never seen the doctor give a report of findings. Never mind. Because the weekly reminders from the consultant usually produce just enough increase in practice income to pay for them. It's a wash!

3. Transfer responsibility. Building on the fear that comes with uncertain times, many doctors are looking for someone to help share the responsibility of running a practice. While the consultant may or may not disclaim this responsibility, for $600 a month, many doctors feel like they're buying someone's attention, expertise, and guiding hand. Like patients who want the doctor to treat their symptoms, doctors often want the management firm to treat the symptoms of

96

their practices. "They're going to help me be successful," muses the doctor. What most doctors overlook is that in the end, it will be themselves who confront patients, fire staff, and give the reports. It's still your practice and your life. Thinking that a consultant will protect you from the future is an illusion. Successful practice is measured by what happens during the course of the doctor/patient relationship.

4. Assume a new debt. There's nothing like a new, large, and recurring expense to get some people motivated! If you don't have the resources to go into debt for a new house or to build a new clinic facility, maybe $600 a month will be enough to get your blood pumping. If you don't have the stomach to ask for referrals, demand perfect compliance from patients, or try out some risky insurance billing procedure, maybe your new monthly obligation will inspire you to do things you don't feel comfortable doing. Debt makes people do all kinds of unsavory things.

5. Get some ideas. Believe it or not, many management firms have a lot of great ideas and have helped thousands of chiropractors implement success habits that have advanced the profession. If you lack a paperwork system, or if you don't have a head for business, or you're just floundering, consider joining. Set yourself a realistic deadline, measurable goals, and disengage after a one-year contract. Implement virtually EVERY procedure, EVERY form, EVERY idea that they teach. Stretch your personality to match that of the firm's namesake. Suppress your inclination to vomit when suggestions are made that conflict with your value system. Allow yourself to be turned into a robot, saying things you don't believe in, and getting patients to do things that are completely outside your comfort zone. After all, it worked for the doctor teaching from the stage. Look where it got him!

Seriously, most of the problems that chiropractors face have little to do with chiropractic. A chiropractic management firm may talk chiropractic lingo and know what buttons to push to get you to join, but the real challenges confronting today's chiropractor are often interpersonal, spiritual, and involve the doctor's personality, self-esteem, and decision-making skills. These are not necessarily chiropractic issues and are rarely addressed successfully in a hotel ball-room with your staff sitting beside you.

Instead of joining a management firm, consider these other alter-natives. Many have been mentioned before by me and others, but they can be effective at getting at the root of the real problem:

1. Read the *E-Myth* by Michael Gerber. He's revised this powerful little book and it's excellent. You won't find the word chiropractic even once, but you'll think he's written a book about your practice. He'll show you the folly of working "in" your practice versus working "on" your practice. True, he offers management consulting services to the small business community, but you can benefit greatly by just reading the book.

2. Study the *Book of Proverbs* in the Bible. The fundamental truths contained in these 31 chapters (read one per day?) are timeless and just as valuable today as when they were written. In fact, after you get out the "good book" you might check out other parts of the Bible explaining the adventures of the world's best healer, leader, and motivator!

3. Get reacquainted with your purpose. Why did you choose chiropractic? If time or money were no object, what would you want to accomplish through your practice of chiropractic? What's standing in the way of producing the "fire in your belly" that got you through chiropractic college? What limitations, barriers, or preconceived notions have you acted upon or allowed to direct your practice away from your original purpose? Who or what is holding you in bondage?

4. Consider counseling. If your's is a control issue, self-esteem issue, fear issue, or personality defect, ask for some help. Simply having the skills to help restore better spinal biomechanics doesn't guarantee that you'll be an effective healer! If a patient presented themselves with the non-chiropractic demons you're battling, what recommendations would you make? Seeking help is not an admit-tance of failure.

5. Team up with a doctor who has a better mind for business. If the business side of chiropractic seems an untamable monster, con-sider hooking up with a doctor who has successfully slayed this

dragon. Maybe he or she wants an associate or would be willing to mentor you with some remedial business advice. You'll discover some incredible insights if you will humble yourself in this way.

Practice should not be a continual struggle. If you haven't experienced the feeling of weightlessness that comes from having your daily experience be in harmony with your mission on this planet, take action. The self-discovery required to take this journey is unlikely to occur while listening to someone else talk about procedures, billing codes, or how they made a million dollars when everyone had $100 deductibles. It cannot be purchased, leased, or taken home on an album of six, 90-minute cassette tapes. Nor are weekly phone calls likely to produce the moments of epiphany we each seek. They can only be obtained by becoming quiet enough, trusting enough, and fearless enough to face ourselves. ■

HOW MUCH
SHOULD I CHARGE?

There is no other subject in chiropractic that can get the hair on the back of a chiropractor's neck to stand at attention than the subject of money. No other topic choreographs the doctor's self-esteem, market sensitivity, business acumen, communication skills, and office protocol in a dance of confusion. Never in the history of chiropractic has patient financial policy been so challenging. And while the following thoughts won't solve this problem, they should give the more open-minded, cutting-edge doctor some ideas to become more confident and resourceful during this time of change.

Certainly, the waters are muddied by the vestiges of indemnity insurance which, when it appears with its high deductibles, is merely catastrophic insurance. Doctors who still harbor sweet memories of abundant $100 deductibles, find acclimating to this change the most difficult. In its place, various types of managed care organizations have sprung up. We have traded heroin for methadone.

Reaping record profits by turning doctors into "providers," lowering reimbursements, minimizing the patient's problem, and generally riding "shotgun" on every doctor's opinion, managed care is often attractively packaged but turns chiropractors into six-visit symptom treaters. Even with the false promise of a continuous stream of patients that never materializes, many chiropractors clamor at the gates, hoping to be included in the local plan. Combine scarcity with a good dose of fear and chiropractors seem willing to sell out their philosophy for the mythical god of security!

Abundant insurance started confusing chiropractors that office visits were actually worth $35, $40, $50 or more. Countless diagnostics and therapeutic devices were implemented solely because insurance policies would pay for them. Some chiropractors soothed their guilty consciences by attending seminars, learning how using these devices could be justified on an analytical basis. Doctors who shunned these money-making schemes were targeted as the cause of professional division and disparaging political bias. They were thought of as fanatical right-wing chiropractors who weren't "scientific" or "modern." It's no surprise that the doctors who never fully embraced the insurance-based practice model are the best at coping with the symptoms of third-party withdrawal.

Time was, chiropractors could call up a half-dozen associates to find out what they were charging and average the figures to set their own rates. That no longer works. Today, "usual and customary" isn't usual or customary! An increasing number of chiropractors recognize that their 1988 insurance-based fee structure won't serve in the "deregulated" practice environment of the 1990s and are wondering what they should be charging their patients.

Before you start tinkering with your fee structure, you need to know how much it costs you to deliver an adjustment. Go back over the last six months or so, and divide your monthly overhead by the number of patient visits you rendered. Include in your overhead the obvious expenses of rent, insurance, and staff salaries, but also your draws and any other recurring expense related to the cost of doing business. This figure tells you how much you need to collect from each visit to tread water by breaking even.

Amazingly, few chiropractors perform this simple arithmetic before offering wellness programs, accepting the fee schedule of a PPO, or making other changes in their financial policy. When they do, they discover the first action step they need to take is to lower their nonessential overhead expenses. Don't throw the baby out with the bath water! The watchwords are "lean and mean." What did you add during the insurance era that may be unnecessary now? Look at every detail from staffing to square footage. Question everything that doesn't directly contribute to serving and educating patients.

The hardest thing for many chiropractors to appreciate is that the services provided in a chiropractic office are not standardized commodities. In the insurance era, an adjustment was an adjustment was an adjustment. That would be like thinking the price of veal scaloppini at Mother Leone's in Manhattan should cost the same as the veal scaloppini served at a Denny's in Boseman, Montana. A lot of factors go into setting the price at both restaurants. Before you fiddle with your fees, recognize that your ability to maintain or even increase your fees is based upon some of the following concerns:

1. Patient education. Without some form of education, patients will never have the opportunity to self-direct their care beyond a shortsighted notion of symptom-relief only. High fees, without patient education is a high stress practice full of symptomatic adults who almost always depend upon third parties for payment. Low fees, without patient education is a frustrating existence in which there is just enough income to survive from month to month. While some patients have no apparent interest in learning about their bodies and the nature of true health, a systematized patient education protocol is a factor in setting fees.

2. Complementing key patient values. What do your patients want to do better or enjoy more when they regain their health? Why is their health important to them? What activity is so valuable to them that they would give up other demands on their income to pay you for chiropractic care? Until you know this valuable information about each patient, your ability to motivate, inspire, and lead them is significantly diminished. Without this knowledge it's tempting to simply offer "cheap" chiropractic care or ascend your soapbox and preach the goodness of a properly functioning nervous system. Your ability to set appropriate fees and more importantly, *collect* your fees, is proportional to your ability to uncover this information and use it in your patient communications.

3. Doctor's personality. Do you have one? Look back to the successful chiropractors before insurance "equality" and you'll see a profession teaming with bold, flamboyant, strong-willed personalities. Who would want to drop $30 with a doctor who is distant, introverted, and uncommunicative? The more interesting the personality, the more the doctor can charge. The better your tableside manners, the more you can charge. The more you can make patients feel good about themselves, the more you can charge. If you're a technique nerd, boorish, or too doctorly, you may find your income diminish in the deregulated world of the post-insurance practice.

4. Staff personality. Don't forget your staff! They often spend more time with the patient than the doctor. A sullen staff member or a front desk assistant on a power trip can debuild a practice in many subtle ways. Patients can quickly tell whether each staff member is on the doctor's team, or merely an employee passing through. Patients look to the staff to be good cheerleaders for chiropractic and to facilitate an optimum experience in the office. Staff members who aren't interesting or interested, detract from the overall office encounter and reduce what a doctor can charge patients.

5. Waiting times. If you ask patients to wait too long, it's difficult to adopt a premium pricing structure. Time is perceived differently by different types of patients. Some come to visit with their friends, others want to get in and out as quickly as possible. Because of this wide range of patient expectations, it's difficult to set a hard and fast rule as to appropriate waiting times. We've all heard the adage "time is money." Until you see your waiting times from your patient's point of view, setting appropriate fees will be difficult.

Office environment, traffic patterns, parking, and other issues need to be considered. The real issue of course, is value. Many patients and doctors get sidetracked into thinking their fee questions are pricing questions, when they are actually value issues. Patients put a different value on their health based upon their education, awareness, socio-economic background, self-esteem, and the other demands on their time and money. Interestingly, every doctor values the chiropractic services they render for the restoration of health in a different way, too.

What do you think you're worth? ∎

PAY NOW
OR PAY LATER

Around the holiday season, everyone from car dealers to department stores advertise some type of delayed payment program. "No interest until April," they purr. "90 days same as cash," they lure. Apparently, the corollary to instant gratification is delayed payment. Examine the budget that congress tries to pass each year and you'll see a similar scenario, only with more zeros. The fact is, the country's budget will be balanced only when we collectively balance our personal budgets. Our governmental representatives are merely reflecting the attitudes of many of their constituents. They will lack the necessary courage to balance the national budget, until we have the courage to put our personal financial houses in order.

There are doctors still looking for a shortcut, or a way to avoid making the sometimes painful choices that must be made. At no other time in recent memory has the desire to "have one's cake and eat it too" become so apparent. Countless doctors have been caught in the glare of the headlights, wanting to keep their fees as high as possible for those rare personal injury and major medical cases, but finding it necessary to keep them low, for those who increasingly find themselves paying cash for chiropractic care. Sound familiar?

For those whose practices are slowly eroding (down as much as 30% from last year), these realizations may be particularly painful. After all, learning that you'll be working harder—for less money, isn't pretty. "What else do you have?" doctors ask, still deep in denial.

"It can't be," they plead, "There's got to be a back door entrance, you know, a 'loophole,'" they whine. "After all, I'm a doctor, and all the research is saying chiropractic is great, you know, and we're more effective than medicine, plus, I still owe money on my huge clinic..."

Take a deep breath... hold... and exhale. It's going to be all right.

While your patient volume may be down, chiropractic works just as well today as it did 100 years ago. Even if your new patient statistics are slumping, there are hundreds, maybe thousands of people who drive by your practice (even right now!) who haven't the foggiest idea who you are or what you do. Meanwhile, you're sitting on your thumbs waiting for the phone to ring. As if great results should speak for itself. As if everyone actually understood and appreciated your unique approach to health. As if anyone cared.

While feeling sorry for yourself, dozens of people in your community are on the operating table getting cut open this very minute. As you sit fixated on yourself, worrying about your accounts payable, hundreds of people within a five mile radius of your office are reaching for their purses, their top desk drawers, or their medicine cabinets to help silence a headache, calm an acidic stomach, or numb some other organ or system. Instead of inventing ways you could better serve, demonstrate your love, and generally "wow" your patients, you're worried about seducing patients you haven't even met yet. Why do you think the universe should entrust you with more patients, if you've dropped the ball with the ones you've been given?

So please, no more, "I'm a victim." No more excuses. No more, "I should haves." No more symptom treating. Today, your practice is the sum total of all the decisions you've made in the past. If you recognize you've made some bad calls, and you're not willing to walk away, then decide this very second to reinvent your practice and get in step with the changing practice climate!

1. Clean out your office. It probably sounds frivolous, based upon the wrenching feeling you're having in your gut, but humor me. It's time to raise your standards and throw out the old stuff that is no longer serving you. Start with your desk. Can you see it? Check your drawers. Are they organized? Fill up a couple of wastebaskets with old journals, professional magazines, and the stuff you set aside to read two years ago. You're going to have to make a lot of decisions about what to keep and what to discard. Make your choices fast. Trust your instinct. When in doubt, toss it! You already have chiropractic figured out, so get rid of the paper ballast that's holding you back.

2. Describe what you want. All too many doctors are waking up after eight or ten years with a practice that barely resembles their original vision. After a decade of opportunity chasing and saluting the every whim of insurance companies, it's time to reclaim your dream. But you've got to be clear about what you want. A vague yearning or a fuzzy, "I'll know it when I see it" won't do. Get a pad of paper and go at it. Your mission is to describe the practice you want, the patients you want, the procedures you want, the staff you want, and the feeling you want, in infinite detail. It must be so vivid, so clear, and so sharp that it becomes real in your mind. How else will you be able to make the right choices to actualize your dream, unless you know what you're trying to create? Describe everything from the shafts of light beaming in through the window, to the giddy feeling you get when you walk in front door. Take your time. Write 20 or 30 pages. Or a book!

3. Get out of your office. If patients aren't showing up in your office, then you don't need to be there! Go visit nearby stores and businesses. Introduce yourself. Hand out as many business cards as possible. Your objective is to get rid of as many business cards as you can. Print five or six different designs. Get to a Toastmasters luncheon. Join some civic groups. Reveal your optimism, excitement about life, and professional pride to as many people as possible. Not feeling optimistic? Then let's start there...

4. Thank your lucky stars! Maybe you've forgotten the huge head start you enjoy in this journey called life because you take your awareness of "cause" for granted. Thank the person who introduced you to chiropractic. Call or write a couple of college professors who influenced your thinking and thank them for their commitment to chiropractic. Write some thank you cards to your favorite patients. Write some letters. Congratulate. Praise. Lift up. Want to be loved? Become a better lover. Want to be appreciated? Be more appreciative.

5. Resume what you already know works. If you've been secretly looking for the "free spinal exam" of the 1980s and coming up empty, let's assume it doesn't exist. In fact, why not just start doing what you already know works? Like running on time. Like educating your patients. Like making chiropractic affordable. Like training your staff. Like making families feel welcome. Like having an office that patients would want to return to again and again. Like being so anxious to anticipate, serve, and exceed your patient's expectations that they'd want to tell the world about you. Too easy? Okay, then if all else fails...

6. Assume the fetal position. The second hundred years of chiropractic may not be your cup of tea. If working harder for less money seems unbecoming, then complete the process of selling out. Find some gullible student, still wet behind the ears, who will pay an inflated price for your trophy case of personal injury and work comp patient files. Yeah, burden some sucker fresh out of school with an overhead that's out of touch with reality and an office that hasn't seen any paint or new carpet in 15 years, and flee. If you got involved in chiropractic for the wrong reason, it's best to make a career change now, after all, the real money is gone. Perfect timing, I might say!

Now, if you're going to stick it out, get cracking. Trim down to your fighting weight and get your dukes up! Patients sucked into managed care need you now, more than ever. Yes, your financial policies probably need a facelift. Rethink your overhead. Simplify your life. Become a chiropractic warrior. Will this be easy? If it was easy, anyone could do it. Which is why so many people are counting on you! ■

COURSE CORRECTIONS

Doctors who ate the rich foods of personal injury cases and the fattening desserts of patients with low insurance deductibles are finding that their dietary habits have bloated their practices and produced hyperlordotic lumbar curves from carrying extra weight around their waists. In retrospect, enjoying these tasty morsels is understandable. The buffet table was continually replenished and virtually every seminar and practice management program taught how to exploit the opportunity presented. After all, everyone was doing it. But times have changed. Some hope that 1986 will return. Others have simply become even more resourceful in ferreting out the increasingly rare cases that have the financial rewards of the past. Still others are misguided into thinking that hospital privileges or acceptance in a sufficient number of managed care organizations is the key to survival. Fortunately, many can read the handwriting on the wall and are professing to repent, embracing the notion of a family based cash practice. And not a minute too soon!

I once worked with a doctor who, besides having a million dollars in tax-free municipal bonds, used a very dictatorial, authoritarian management style with his four associate-run clinics. Associate doctors and staff members lived in constant fear of losing their jobs. Information about the health and direction of the business was kept secret. Surprise visits, and new instructions barked over brief phone calls, interrupted the care of patients. As I saw staff members of this organization emotionally disengaged and doctors merely contributing the bare minimum to keep their jobs, I decided my mission was to change the management approach of this self-made millionaire.

I might as well have wanted to single-handedly clear up the national debt or bring permanent peace to Bosnia!

Like the alcoholic who must first hit bottom before being available for, and acting on, the suggestion of sobriety, so it was with this doctor. While his practices weren't what they could be, they were "successful" in the traditional sense, so why change?

That's not the problem with the many doctors who recognize the game has changed. They quickly admit that they should've, could've, would've (educated their patients, saved more of their money, etc.), and freely admit they "blew it." Now, they want to respond to the changes and have the cash-based wellness practice of their dreams.

And they want it now!

Talk to the captains who pilot the big super oil tankers across the Atlantic or the navigators who push heavy barges up the Mississippi River. These massive chunks of real estate are sluggish. Making course corrections requires taking action many miles in advance. The momentum of these crafts makes it difficult to stop quickly or make quick turns to avoid hazards—not unlike the predicament a doctor faces when a change in their practice style is required.

The first strategy is to tap the trophy case of inactive work comp and personal injury patient files. However, your attempts at reactivation fall on deaf ears, because while grateful for the symptomatic results you produced when insurance paid the fee, these patients don't understand chiropractic. Because these worker's compensation patients see wellness care as a needless luxury, they are not inclined to revisit your office until they slip and fall or get rear-ended again. Because educating those personal injury cases seemed like an unnecessary waste, they are not inclined to return and pay for their care out of their own pockets. The fact is, you had a promotion, not a practice; an acute care center, not a health care facility; you were treating a policy, not a patient.

The sad truth is, you're starting over.

Not unlike the new graduate looking for the first new patients, countless doctors with established practices and ten years or more of excellent clinical results, are waking up to find their practices have vanished. Either by a sudden limitation on PIP coverage in their state, insurance reform, or the installation of gatekeepers in the work comp structure, the health of lots of practices changed overnight. It is only from this vantage point that the carrot dangled by managed care organizations must seem palatable. Clinging to the scraps of flotsam and jetsam from the 1980s with a clammy death grip, all too many doctors are going from the frying pan into the fire. Remember, managed care is about management, not about care!

While many doctors who find themselves in this predicament resent the obvious solutions, and would rather avoid expending the energy required to restart their practices, here are some ways to jump-start a plateaued practice:

1. Public speaking. This is probably the most sophisticated and effective way to restart a practice. Sure, the instant gratification of coupons and mailings is missing, but it's a great way to reveal your values, personality, and experience. Right this very minute, the program directors for countless civic groups and service organizations are pulling their hair, wondering who they can get next month to entertain the "troops" over a rubber chicken lunch. Solve their problem! Outreach programs, in which you get to share your unique view of health and human physiology, pay off by trusting the audience to do the right thing when they feel it is appropriate.

2. Influence the influencers. Make a list of the small businesses in your immediate area that see lots of people every day. At the top of your list make sure you include the beauticians, dry cleaners, travel agents, and similar businesses that tend to influence the behavior of others. Target these businesses with a regular appearance. Start frequenting them, even if that means spreading your dry cleaning around among three establishments! Give the cosmetologists, insurance agents, and waitresses in your vicinity something to talk about: you!

3. Conduct patient focus groups. Arrange to meet five or six patients for lunch at a nearby restaurant. Ask them questions about what they like and don't like about the practice, the procedures, the staff, the parking; that sort of thing. Your job is to uncover ways the office can offer better service to the kinds of patients you'd especially enjoy serving.

4. Identify your ideal patient. Again, it sounds so unproductive at a time when you need anyone warmer than room temperature in the practice. However, it's easy to wake up years from now, trapped in a practice with patients you don't like. Can you and your staff recognize the types of patients you want to rebuild your practice with? How do they think? How do they pay? What kind of car do they drive? Do they have children?

5. Work out. You probably need to get back down to fighting weight after enjoying all those high cholesterol foods from the insurance era. Plan to give yourself 20 to 30 minutes of vigorous physical exercise every day. Increase your lung capacity and the health of your cardiovascular system. Get ready to handle the demand for your unique and highly-effective approach to health care.

6. Read non-chiropractic books. Since you've got chiropractic figured out now, the remaining uncharted territory is how to think like the types of patients you want to attract to your practice. Read some books outside of chiropractic! My favorites are *The E-Myth* by Michael Gerber, *How to Win Customers and Keep Them For Life* by Michael LeBoeuf, Ph.D., *Customers For Life* by Carl Sewell, *Marketing Without Advertising* by Michael Phillips and Salli Rasberry, and *Positively Outrageous Service* by T. Scott Gross.

"But Bill, I need new patients now!" Remember how you tell patients that they've had the problem for quite a while and it's going to take time to see improvement? Same thing here. Remember how you warn some patients that their problem may actually get worse, before it gets better? Same thing here. Remember the alcoholic who has to hit bottom before seeking help and making change? Same thing here. ■

WALKING THE LINE

Unlike manufacturing, in which products are produced, in professions like dentistry or chiropractic, services are performed. The chiropractic "performance" encompasses much more than a thorough examination and a perfectly rendered adjustment. In fact, the clinical aspects of the chiropractic performance are expected as part of the "package", in the same way we expect the stage performance of a rock band to include guitars and drums. And while the musicians may have a specific preference for a particular manufacturer of guitars, or brand of drums, the subtle differences are lost on the screaming fans in the audience.

It's interesting that what doctors think is important, is often unimportant to patients, and what doctors see as unimportant, is often a very high priority among patients!

This perceptual difference produces something that is rarely discussed and which tends to cloud the doctor/patient relationship. After years of schooling, assuming a huge debt, referring to oneself as "doctor," and taking on the social responsibility (and privileges) of being a doctor, you are still a service provider. Sure, there may be more prestige and importance attached to being a doctor than, say, a waitress, brick layer, or an insurance salesman, but in the end, all are service providers. Servants.

Serving others is among the highest callings, and helping the hurting masses as a doctor is a special calling. However, embracing one's role as a servant, recognizing that one's "master" is a sniffling parade of myopic, idiosyncratic patients who are ignorant about chiro-practic can be disconcerting!

Doctors who chaff at this realization and recognize that in the final analysis the patient controls the doctor patient relationship, create a variety of coping schemes to cover, or at least ameliorate the problem. Which strategy do you use?

My way or the highway. This doctor/patient model can be as extreme as dismissing patients who don't keep their appointments or denying care to those who won't attend "Wednesday-evening-special-appointment-spinal-care-workshop-lectures." It may be as subtle as a policy that forbids staff members from discussing fees over the telephone with a prospective patient.

This strategy is based upon a form of intimidation. By denying access to chiropractic, or even withdrawing care by forcing patients to accept, appreciate, or salute some obscure procedure or belief, or to deify the doctor, are some of the most extreme examples used by doctors compensating for their low self-esteem and who wish to create the illusion of being in control. When this leadership style is combined with perfectionistic tendencies, only the patients who are the easiest to control, find the office hospitable. They refer friends with a similar lack of discernment, reaffirming the doctors iron-fisted approach to patient control, creating a self-fulfilling prophecy.

Solution: Careful! This dictatorial management style is out of date and is no longer as effective as it once was. Lighten up a little. Remember, when patients agree to become patients, they're not asking you to become their conscience or assume the role of den mother. Pride comes before the fall. Have another slice of humble pie.

Hit me. Beat me. Make me write bad checks. At the opposite end of the spectrum is the doctor who annually wins the chiropractic wimp award. Here, the inmates are running the asylum, because the doctor lacks the ability to confront patients and the self-esteem necessary to endure patient (or staff) criticism. The doctor so badly wants to be liked and accepted by the patient, that he or she is willing to minimize the patient's problem, "forget" to tell patients ways to avoid their problem, or even to demand payment for services!

These pathetic creatures thrived during the insurance era when the only confrontational skills required was the ability to hire staff members who could call insurance companies all day long. Cash-paying patients were, well, a bother. At least with a sugar daddy insurance policy, you could focus on clinical concerns and not have to get your hands "dirty" by discussing financial matters.

Those days are gone. Today, as these doctors crawl out from underneath their rocks, rubbing their eyes in the bright sunshine, they are finding practice more difficult. New patient statistics are down, collections are down, and the staff is nervously wondering about the future.

Solution: Short of a personality transplant, if you find yourself facing this Rip Van Winkle challenge, consider taking action steps to shed your lack of confrontational tolerance. Join a toastmasters group. Force yourself into some risky situations. Consider a "work hardening" program that can fortify your self-confidence and fragile ego. Assume a leadership position in your chiropractic association or society. Look for ways to "take a few arrows" by standing up for your beliefs. If you don't know what you believe, start a journal. Articulate your beliefs, your philosophy, and world view so you'll always know where you stand on everything from first visit adjusting to immunizations and everything in between. And remember, you chose chiropractic—a profession most people don't understand, don't like, don't think works, and don't think is necessary. Why do you expect to be liked in the first place?

Pass the buck to a third party. Some doctors are so uncomfortable with the ambiguity of the doctor/patient relationship and their role as servants, they'd rather look to the government or some managed care organization to clarify or adjudicate the relationship.

Here, the doctor has surrendered his or her freedom in exchange for "security" or the illusion of objectivity. It's simply more convenient to accept the statistical "science" of a symptomatic treatment protocol rather than have to justify or persuade patients of the value of the chiropractic lifestyle *they* enjoy. Avoiding the controversy of adjusting newborns, underage children, or recommending wellness care, turns chiropractic into a mere biomechanical procedure; a natural, drug-free, low-tech therapy for low back pain. This is security? It sounds like imprisonment!

Third parties interfere in the doctor/patient relationship. Whether it's an attorney, a bureaucrat, a statistician, or the government. When other agendas get superimposed, the outcome is rarely in the best interest of the patient.

Solution: Enlarge your vision of chiropractic. If you find yourself trapped in the windowless room of symptom treating, personal injury cases, and feel the heavy thumb of managed care, plan your escape! Track down some colleagues who have family practices, who regularly see newborns, who have patients who pay cash because they understand and value chiropractic. Get to a pediatric seminar. Discover ways to associate each patient's key values or interests (family, golf, gardening, etc.) with benefits that can be derived by chiropractic care. Take a self-inventory of your own motives for regular chiropractic checkups. Wouldn't virtually every patient benefit from a similar visit schedule?

Grow better patients. A famous men's clothing store in New York claims that "our best customer is an informed customer." Their strategy is to create more discerning customers who can understand, appreciate, and value the sometimes subtle differences among different types of seemingly similar men's suits. The same strategy can work in chiropractic, too.

The media is not a friend of chiropractic. The hospitals and established medical industrial complex are not friends of chiropractic. Insurance companies and other third parties are not friends of chiropractic. The only potential supporters of chiropractic are the millions of patients who have benefited over the years. Unfortunately, many of these patients are not the referral ambassadors and chiropractic advocates they could be. Lacking consistent, effective patient education, chiropractic is merely something that "happened" to them. Like the sterile mule, they can't replicate themselves, stunting the growth and acceptance of chiropractic.

Educated patients are the best security blanket. Educated patients ask better questions, make better decisions, are better equipped to defend their chiropractic decision, and are more likely to tell others.

Solution: I'm often asked at seminars if there is a common problem or issue that comes up in the patient focus groups I've conducted. The most common observation is the total lack of understanding that even the doctor's very best patients exhibit. If you haven't inspired a patient or two in the last year to go to chiropractic college, then you have a ways to go in your patient education efforts.

Education is the way servants can create better masters. ■

THE MASTER
AND THE SERVANT

As a child, I was often asked to assist my Dad in various projects around the house. For several years my Dad was a woodworker, building and installing kitchen cabinets. He was very handy and used these skills to remodel our home. His workshop was in the basement. When he needed help cutting, gluing, or nailing, he would often call my Mom or my brother or I, for the assistance of a second pair of hands. As my brother and I got older, we would increasingly replace our Mom as his assistant and the demands made upon us to hold, guide, or measure something increased.

As youngsters, our inability to read our Dad's mind proved to be a serious obstacle. Because we didn't know or appreciate the objectives, difficulties, or purpose of what Dad was trying to do, we invariably pointed the flashlight in the wrong place, held the board at the wrong angle, or performed some other task with less than adequate sufficiency. Our shortcomings were quickly pointed out at several decibels above normal conversation and caused both my brother and I to be only reluctant assistants.

While a patient rarely raises his or her voice, they express their displeasure with the assistance they receive from their chiropractor in other ways. The fact is, the doctor/patient partnership is a classic example of the servant/master relationship. Unlike the teaching of some practice consultants, the patient is the master and the doctor is the servant. Ignoring this fundamental truth or employing procedures or policies that attempt to reverse these roles, either backfires or tends to diminish the potential of the practice.

Much of the training that today's young doctors receive, tends to obliterate this helpful metaphor governing the doctor/patient relationship. Walk down the halls of any chiropractic college and you can often tell which students are in the early stages of their indoctrination and which ones are close to assuming their rightful position in society as doctors. The former look like students at any other college, and the latter have started to dress and act the part.

The prestige and social standing afforded doctors, (while less today then 20 years or more ago) helps confuse this important issue. "Act like the doctor you are," commands the school clinic director. Suddenly, the person, who just a year or two earlier was outgoing and approachable, assumes an aloof, omniscient, doctorly persona that more and more satisfaction surveys suggest that patients don't like. In the process, the young doctor forgets that he or she is the servant, and the patient is the master.

But patients don't deserve to be the master, you argue. They are weak, in pain, and lack the understanding and wisdom of true health. This inequality further obscures the servant/master relationship. We rarely think of servants being more powerful than their master. This is the same principle that creates the hubris surrounding politicians sent to Washington or even the capricious local building inspector. They are supposed to be our servants, yet often their own agendas or a craving for power, blinds them to this simple fact. Perhaps the most memorable example of this was U.S. Congressman Tom Foley who sued the citizens of Washington state when they tried to impose term limits!

What makes a good servant? If you take your role as a servant seriously, you might consider a review of the Bible. It contains countless guidelines on the conduct and behavior of servants. Perhaps these observations will give you some ideas on ways you can enhance the respect and appreciation you receive from your masters!

1. Multiply the master's resources. One of my favorite parables in the *New Testament* is the story about the talents. In biblical times, talents were a form of wealth or currency. If you remember, a property owner (the master) left his property in the charge of three of his servants, giving them various numbers of talents for safekeeping while he was gone. Upon his return he discovered one servant had invested his talents, multiplying them into three, another into ten, and the remaining servant safely produced the same talent that had been entrusted to him. The Bible tells us that the servant who had done nothing to grow the value of the talent he had been given, received a stern lecture! Apparently, servants are expected to nurture, enlarge, and improve that which they have been given custody.

What does that mean in a chiropractic setting? Perhaps it means that doctors are to demonstrate ways the patient can save money, get well faster, and avoid a relapse in the future. Maybe it means that doctors must give patients more than they paid for. Simply making each patient more valuable, by improving their self worth would be a significant accomplishment. Yet, few doctors risk venturing into the emotional and spiritual domains required to produce this type of response. Instead, most doctors prefer the shallow end of the pool, limiting their patient relationships to merely the physical and the biomechanical. Literally burying their hidden talent in the process, patients leave the office with exactly what they brought—except their physical complaint has been alleviated. The very best servants add value.

2. Work hard with a cheerful spirit. The attitude in which service is rendered may be one of the most important aspects of extraordinary service. Tired of the seemingly unappreciative customers, many sales clerks, shoe salesmen, and hair stylists reveal their apparent disdain for their customers in subtle ways. Countless doctors and staff members are guilty of acting as their job would somehow be nirvana—if it just weren't for patients! Often, the patient is perceived as the problem. "It would be a great business—if it weren't for those &@#?%! patients."

How many times have you been on the receiving end of a waitresses' first night on the job or the robotically-slurred speech of two junior high school students selling something door-to-door to raise money for a school project? By any conventional standard their furtive efforts of providing service were pathetic. But their attitude, their desire to serve, their ambition, and their bright-eyed enthusiasm more than overcame their lack of experience or ineptitude.

Attitude reveals the true intentions of the servant. The servant who is anxious to please is not only rare, he or she is more often given the benefit of the doubt. Sure, their tip jar is fuller, but in the case of a doctor, the right attitude is virtually an inoculation against accusations of malpractice and a virtual new patient and referral magnet. Attitude can't be faked (we can detect a false "Miss America" smile). Attitude can't be compensated for by an incredible adjusting technique or high tech diagnostics. Attitude is that "extra special something" that separates average doctors, from those who are growing in spite of the pressures from managed care. God loves a cheerful giver.

Serving others is the highest calling any of us render. Each of us is rewarded in direct proportion to our service to others and the value we add to the universe. Through chiropractic, doctors and staff members have enormous opportunities to be of service. With refined acuity, these opportunities can be identified in other areas beyond the physical complaints that prompt patients to seek out your services. Apparently, the way you master chiropractic is to become a better servant. ■

TALK WALKING

Perhaps one of the most profound joys of a lifetime is raising children. Some might rate their other accomplishments as more important or more financially rewarding, but nurturing a child's development and launching them as responsible citizens may be the most satisfying endeavors. Not only are we creating a legacy, but we have the opportunity to correct "the mistakes" of *our* parents. Remember vowing as a teenager that when you become a parent you weren't going to do such and such to your child? It's not until we hear our 4-year old parrot some of our less-than-desirable language or see our 5-year old mimicking an embarrassing personal habit that we discover the full implications of being a parent. This is when we grow in our respect and appreciation for our own parents. It is also the moment when we discover an overlooked aspect of patient motivation.

While considerable thought is given to primary school curriculum and the pros and cons of phonics, "new math", and outcome based education, the most significant type of learning occurs in the home. The values and examples set by parents, relatives, and other trusted role models make an inestimable contribution to child development. Children use their unblinking X-ray vision and built-in tape recorders to document our every movement, every attitude, every intonation, and every value-laden decision. Many times an uncensored or off-handed remark has come back to haunt us, blushing as we hear our child repeat it in an inappropriate context. In the same way children learn by example, so do many patients. We look to the values, behaviors, commitment, and passion of our doctors for valuable clues in directing our conduct and response to the doctor's recommendations. So it shouldn't come as any surprise that many doctors have created an entire practice of patients who look for short-term solutions and avoid making the commitment so necessary for optimum results. Like patients who don't want true health, but instead opt for merely feeling better, countless doctors have no higher goal than to pay the bills.

1. Maintenance care. One of the most obvious and seemingly easiest incongruencies between some doctors and the expectations they have of their patients is the chiropractic care *they* receive. Incredibly, many chiropractors neglect their own health and fail to regularly obtain the maintenance care they beg their patients to embrace. This discrepancy is even more ironic in the face of the often unlimited access most chiropractors have to care that is free and can be obtained without having to cool their heels in a crowded reception room at 5:30 PM.

Action step: Just as a lawyer who represents himself has a fool for a client, take your own chiropractic care more seriously. Have the doctor you receive your care from work you up like a "real" patient. Commit to a program of care that is relevant to your lifestyle. Become a model patient yourself.

2. Family care. The dirty little secret in many chiropractic households is that the doctor's children often go without chiropractic care! Like the cobbler's children who go shoeless, many children of chiropractors go without chiropractic care. Ironically, the reverse is often true, too. Doctors who claim they don't treat their patient's symptoms are often at home adjusting their children at the drop of a hat for everything from cranky bedtime behavior to a dislike for green beans. Certainly chiropractors aren't the only ones who suffer from a double standard; however when you recognize how difficult it is to practice what you preach, you might be inclined to be more understanding with the demands you place on your patients.

Action step: Just as it is difficult to be a prophet in your home town, it's easy for your own family to lose respect for chiropractic. Avoid dishonoring chiropractic by subverting it in your own family.

You may need a set of travel cards at the office and one at home, but start taking the incredible power of chiropractic more seriously with your own family and you'll discover your family of patients will take it more seriously, too.

3. Opportunity chasing. When doctors start losing faith in chiropractic, they often start looking for other income building schemes. As they take their eyes off their patients needs and investigate the personal rewards of multi-level marketing ideas or other diversions, patients lose faith in chiropractic as well. As doctors "hedge their bets" with excursions into everything from ostrich farming to enzyme supplements, patients are less willing to put all of their health care "eggs" into the single basket of chiropractic. So they maintain a supply of aspirin, keep the prescription handy in case they may need it, and get their children inoculated anyway. If the doctor's going to have a lucky rabbit's foot, the patient wants one too.

Action step: Retake your chiropractic vows. Either you believe chiropractic has value, or you don't. And just because insurance deductibles have soared and the monster of managed care seems to be hiding behind every bush, it doesn't mean chiropractic has lost its simplicity, efficacy, or cost effectiveness. Nor does it mean that patients no longer benefit like they used to. In fact from what I hear, the exact opposite is true.

4. Out of shape. While this is somewhat related to the first issue raised above, it has a more subtle affect. Even with a regular schedule of wellness chiropractic care, many chiropractors have neglected other more obvious aspects of their health. Some still smoke. Even more are noticeably overweight. And many others don't regularly floss their teeth or practice many of the other simplest health maintenance habits. Patients often notice these "imperfections" and find the doctor's chiropractic recommendations hollow or unbelievable. Patients rarely take their health more seriously than their doctor.

Action step: Of course the solution is obvious. Setting an example with your overall picture of health can become a compelling testimonial for your patients. Admit your shortcomings and make a serious commitment to set some new, healthier habits. If you need to lose some weight, become accountable by informing your staff. Take before and after pictures. Offer hope for patients who need to slay the same dragons.

5. Late to office. You can always tell how much fun doctors are having by whether they show up on time for their first patient. Not only does this set a bad example for the staff, but patients sense that the doctor isn't really interested in them. Besides not honoring the patient's time, the doctor is rarely "centered" and able to respond to the more subtle needs of their first couple of patients. In fact, it is a doctor's ability to recognize and tend to these psychological, spiritual, and emotional needs that separate the average doctor from the extraordinary—something unlikely to occur if you're out of breath and still smelling of toast and coffee.

Action step: Be the first one in the office. Set a good example. One doctor I know comes in early to "practice" seeing patients! He'll go into each adjusting room, pretend to greet the patients, adjust them, and perform his other clinical routines. By the time his staff and first patient shows up he is focused and ready to serve. No wonder he has such busy mornings.

6. Doctors not excited about chiropractic. More and more doctors I meet either take chiropractic for granted, or are frustrated by the control they seem to be losing to third parties. Doctors who have turned their destinies over to the cost-cutting moods of managed care organizations or the whims of government bureaucrats who don't even understand chiropractic, are getting what they deserve. Doctors who are waking up to the fact that an overdependence upon third parties has turned their honorable careers into a high-risk job, have become disillusioned. Patients can sense this increasing bitterness. They may not be aware of its cause, so many suspect that *they* are the source of the doctor's unhappiness! The result is a practice that begins a downward spiral and ironically, becomes seemingly more dependent upon third parties.

Action step: Remember, patients are rarely more excited about chiropractic than the doctor and staff. It may require an Oscar-winning performance on your part, but you'd better bring the passion

126

back into your chiropractic act! The patient isn't the problem. It's your inability to sufficiently communicate and demonstrate the value of chiropractic. If the patient is in the clutches of a short-sighted-money-hungry-claims-cutting HMO, your patient is the real victim, not you! Keep a stiff upper lip. When you give up, you dash a patient's hope—critical to the patient's respect, recovery, and referrals.

Next to making mistakes and learning the hard way, the second most effective way we learn is by the example set by those around us. Videos, brochures, reports, and even lectures have their place, but the example set by doctors and their staff can have even more influence. The "do-as-I-say, not-as-I-do" school of patient motivation was never that effective. Maybe we think we're covering up our own shortcomings by pointing to a mythical or philosophical ideal. But like children who rebel as teenagers when they discover the inconsistencies of their parents behaviors, patients often drop out and become a statistic to a doctor's inability or unwillingness to set a good example. ■

THE ONE NIGHT STAND

This moment in time you're experiencing right now is the result of a lifetime of decisions. I am glad your decisions led you to this opportunity for me to share some ideas. These ideas may stimulate you to make some new decisions that, hopefully, will serve to reinforce and nurture your life spirit.

As we go about the task of making choices, everything from taking that second helping of pie, to who we have chosen to spend our lives with is the result of our decision-making powers. The ability to differentiate, express a preference, and decide, is how we take steps in our journey to a destination that we never reach. Our decision to feel insulted when someone questions our validity, or to feel exhilarated by a glorious sunrise are merely choices that we each freely make—usually without thinking. Our conditioned responses often trap us in a rut, which may explain why so many chiropractors find themselves on a treadmill, held hostage by debt, lack of discipline, fear, patients, staff members, managed care organizations, insurance companies, lawyers, or a lack of new patients.

Ironically, based upon the care most chiropractors choose for their families and themselves, they've already had enough new patients. Their challenge is not a lack of new patients, it's the inability to *keep* patients!

Seems to me that if you embrace the notion of looking beyond a patient's symptoms for the cause of a patient's health complaint, then some type of continuing maintenance/wellness/preventive chiropractic care makes sense. Waiting for the occurrence of a subjective complaint before taking action would be like waiting for an automobile accident to occur before buckling one's seat belt. If nothing else, with the limitation of matter and the irreversibility of certain disease states, waiting for obvious symptoms to appear ignores the nature of true intelligence—the ability to adapt.

The decision to take the path of least resistance and become fixated on a constant search for new patients, at the expense of shepherding existing patients, feeds the fear that many chiropractors are experiencing during this time of change. And why not? After all, chiropractic colleges don't teach courses entitled "Patient Retention 101" or a 9th trimester class called "Essentials of Client Relationships." No, instead the focus is entirely on sick people. People whose personalities are distorted by pain, whose outlooks are short term, and who are easiest to manage and control. The result is a whole generation of chiropractors who have become biomechanical nerds, structural engineers, or symptom-treaters interested in hospital privileges, third party reimbursement, and "acceptance."

It starts like a blind date. The anticipation of meeting a new patient must be intoxicating. The pulse quickens, the adrenalin pumps, and a sense of increased awareness overcomes the body as you prepare to meet your next chiropractic "conquest." After settling into the accepted social pleasantries, the tension diminishes as your practiced routine takes over, delivering your introductory "pick up" lines at the consultation with practiced professionalism.

While you can hardly wait to get your hands on him/her, you must not move too quickly, lest they get the wrong idea! Some rush in on the first visit, others resist the temptation and wait until the second get-together. Fortunately, most patients embrace chiropractic and respond warmly.

Like the early stages of romantic involvement, you can hardly wait to see each other. You smile when you see the name on the appointment book. During this early stage of the relationship you spend lots of time together, promising to call if there's ever a problem. As you lavish time and attention, the patient rewards you with praise as his or her symptomatic picture improves. The relationship is hot!

When it seems the patient has embraced chiropractic, marriage is proposed. The ceremony is brief and the honeymoon is often post-poned. Meanwhile, you find yourself more interested in the other members of the wedding party. Suddenly, the flowers and candy and dreamy-eyed philosophical discussions are abandoned. The passion has evaporated into dull, routine visits. You've lost interest. Anyway, there's someone new in your life. It's a low back case with some interesting systemic problems...

How many times do you need to prove to yourself that chiropractic works? How many times do you have to put your diagnostic skills and adjusting technique to the test to have the assurance that it's effective? Why the short term vision?

While the following ideas may not produce the heart-pounding rush that getting your hands on a new patient offers, here are some ideas that can make long term patient relationships more fulfilling:

1. Identify your current chiropractic clients. The word "client" comes the Latin word meaning to "lean on." The word "patient" means "to suffer." After patients are no longer suffering, they often leave. Have you ever thought about the "non-suffering" portion of your current practice? Do you have one? And perhaps more impor-tantly, what is there about you, your tableside manner, or your office environment that would prompt a patient to want to remain as a client? If obvious symptoms motivated them to investigate your services, what are you offering to replace that source of motivation?

List the names of currently active patients who seem to have embraced a chiropractic lifestyle. These are patients who are probably paying cash and show up anywhere from once a month or so, to two and three times a month. Try to identify common traits; anything from their age, whether they have children, to whether they drive foreign built automobiles or hold white collar jobs. If you want more of these types of people, find out what makes them tick and why chiropractic seemingly "took" for them, but not for the countless other patients you've helped. The more you know about the personalities, lifestyles, interests, attitudes, and desires of your current lifestyle patients, the more easily you'll be able to attract and keep similarly-minded patients.

2. Compute the lifetime value of a patient. If the profitability of new patients, with the expensive examinations and X-rays turns your head, maybe you're thinking too short term. If your typical case average is around $1000, including exams, X-rays, and 20 to 30 visits that are spread out over 90 days or so, how long would it take to exceed that same figure by adjusting that same patient just once a month? Two or three years? With virtually zero marketing costs and the distracting and productivity-stunting non-clinical tasks required of new patients gone, your practice is more focused and efficient. "Collect" enough of these types of patients and you have an HMO-proof practice in which you can laugh at yellow page salesmen and enjoy regular vacations.

Doctors who already recognize the value of creating long-term relationships with their patients can inadvertently undermine their chances by pushing too hard. Using the dating metaphor earlier, if you talk about your previous romantic involvements or discuss marriage and children too soon, you can scare off your prospect! Don't take the inevitable rejection personally or make patients feel like losers because they don't fit your model of optimum patient behavior. Instead, think of each new patient as the beginning of a 20 or 30 year relationship that may be punctuated by long periods of absence. Make reactivations a time of celebration and rejoicing. Keep in touch. Assume mutual respect.

Like the sexually transmitted diseases of the sexual revolution, the chiropractic version of the one-night stand has left behind a legacy of bloated doctor lifestyles with atrophied communication skills. The question more doctors should be asking themselves, is whether patients will "respect them in the morning." And by the looks of all too many offices with the trophy cases of inactive patient files and empty reception rooms, the answer seems pretty clear. ■

EARLY WARNING SYSTEM

About the time I was learning how to protect myself in the event of a nuclear attack by climbing under my school desk, my *Weekly Reader* explained something called the DEW Line. No, it had nothing to do with the water droplets clinging to the grass in the morning. It was an acronym for some joint U.S. and Canadian project that consisted of an array of big electronic dishes which constantly monitored the horizon for incoming nuclear missiles. Thanks to these high-tech listening posts along the Arctic Circle, students like us would have an additional 50 minutes of warning before the blinding flash of light and we were vaporized. This constant monitoring and increased sensitivity is similar to the heightened awareness that chiropractors have about their personal health. It gives doctors a distinct advantage over patents, prompting most to adopt some type of ongoing wellness/preventive chiropractic care. For some, this may entail daily checks. For others, once every two or three months seems enough. Why is it so difficult to motivate patients to adopt a similar "chiropractic lifestyle"?

Unless a chiropractor has bought into a medical model of chiropractic, leaning towards a six visit, non-invasive treatment for low back pain (at least there *is* research that proves chiropractic works for *that*!), many chiropractors yearn for a stable, cash practice of appreciative families enjoying regular, non-symptomatic wellness care. Is this merely a pipe dream or some unattainable vision advanced by seminar lecturers? Perhaps. The reality of anything even close, is dependent upon more chiropractors recognizing why this is so rare, and discerning what can be done to find a close approximation to this stress-free way of practice. Doctors and patients look at health from two very different points of view.

Doctors value their health. The difficultly in getting patients to adopt a chiropractic lifestyle isn't because patients don't have a clue as to the value of maintenance care. Just look at the way some patients baby their cars! They have their oil changed religiously every 3,000 miles. They have them washed once a week. The fact is, many patients value their cars more than their own health. More telling is that they purchase the most prestigious cars they can afford, and then abandon them three years later and get a new one! The only hope in helping patients value something that they currently don't value, is a relentless patient education program that makes chiropractic relevant.

Why doctors are doctors. What causes some people to become welders and others to become doctors is a mystery. Probably one of the things that attracted you to chiropractic was how it affirmed your own outlook on health. One's health consciousness is something formed at an early age and heavily influenced by our parents. For the very reason you're interested in health matters, you have an advantage over the patient whose attention turns to health concerns only at the site of blood, or when an entire limb goes numb. This increased awareness makes it difficult, maybe impossible, to fully appreciate the limited interest patients have in health issues.

Doctors are focused on health. While a doctor's life revolves around health issues, patients have other concerns. Patients have hobbies, work interests, friends who aren't involved in health care, financial concerns, and all the other minutia that accompanies modern life. Instead of living for the chance of having a perfect spine, most patients merely want their health to be a non-issue. The only time their health seems to matter is when their *lack* of health gets in the way. Most people rarely appreciate the importance of their automobiles until they break down. Same with most peoples' health. It only garners attention when it is gone. The only hope of encouraging patients to continue with care beyond a "first aid" approach to relief care, is to associate chiropractic with something each patient enjoys or values when they are healthy.

Doctors know too much. Doctors who have seen actual cholesterol plaque attached to an artery wall, the stringy scar tissue in muscles, and the dirty lungs of a smoker who is now a cadaver, have an unfair advantage. A doctor's training equips you with dramatic, overpowering evidence of the ramifications of certain health choices. It gives many doctors the discipline to avoid red meat, shy away from coffee, swear off milk, or take a stand on a dozen other issues that most patients rarely even think about. Because patients in a chiropractic office are rarely exposed to anything with the impact of human dissection, they aren't inclined to fully appreciate the consequences of their decisions.

Doctors have more confidence. It isn't long before chiropractors have had just about everything walk through their front door. After a couple of years in practice, there aren't too many surprises left. By then, most doctors have helped enough patients to feel confident about their technique, clinical skills, and the need to trust the inborn healing ability that patients bring with them when they begin care. Most patients are never told, "You represent my 235th headache case" or "You'll be receiving my 750,000th safely delivered adjustment." In most cases, the doctor is much more confident about the successful outcome than patients. For patients consulting your office it's often their last hope. For you, it's just business as usual.

Doctors become disinterested. Many doctors are quick to tell their patients that they can't judge their health by their symptoms, yet as soon as the patient is symptom-free, many of these same doctors lose interest in the patient! Apparently it is more emotionally satisfying for doctors to see symptoms disappear (chiropractic works!), even though they don't want their patients to use their symptoms as a guide for the necessity for continued care. With the symptoms gone, visits degenerate into long periods of waiting, while time-consuming sick patients are seen, followed by a brief and superficial visit in which the doctor scolds patients about their weight, their continued smoking, or previously missed appointments. If patients are to pay for this type of care out their own pockets, then in most offices, the emotional, psychological, and social benefits of seeking continued chiropractic care needs to be reconsidered from the patient's point of view.

Doctors don't pay for their care. Let's not overlook the obvious! It's easy for doctors to act on their own early warning system of impending health needs because there are few financial consequences to getting a chiropractic "tune-up." At the earliest notification; a sniffle, a sore throat, a headache—chiropractors can head down the street for a free chiropractic adjustment. They don't have to give up eating out tonight, a movie with the family, or reprioritize any other financial matters. Frankly, it costs patients money to be too aware of their health! Instead, most patients simply wait until the need for care is more pressing.

It's essential if doctors are going to understand patients, and have appropriate expectations of them, that they take these issues into consideration. It's the same shock we have upon discovering someone who doesn't like our favorite food or share our musical tastes.

This challenge is likely to continue until the chiropractic profession makes a concerted effort to change health attitudes among elementary school-aged children. The doctors who enjoy the second hundred years of this profession will benefit from your efforts to present chiropractic principles in classrooms. Health attitudes are slow to change, but they *do* change. They are easier to create in children, than change in adults. And with the threat of nuclear annihilation reduced these days, maybe it's time chiropractic was represented in the pages of the *Weekly Reader*! ∎

YOU WERE RIGHT!

A major medical teaching university has just announced that it will begin teaching chiropractic alongside medical treatments. While some embrace this development with pride and acceptance, historians may someday remember this date as the beginning of the end of chiropractic as we know it.

With the positive results bound to accrue from teaching chiropractic approaches, it isn't hard to imagine a full-fledged "Physical Medicine" department at teaching universities, hospitals, and traditional medical facilities. Before long, with excellent results with neuromuscular-skeletal complaints, it's easy to imagine someone suggesting that physical medicine techniques (chiropractic terms will be quickly replaced) might work with other health problems besides headaches and low back pain. "Let's test it and find out!" After generally positive results, spinal manipulation becomes mainstream and is considered the first treatment of choice before resorting to drug therapy or surgical intervention. Finally, we got what we wanted. Didn't we?

What's more important, chiropractic philosophy—or the results that chiropractic-like care produces? What's more important, intention or results? What's more important, your job as a chiropractor or that millions more who might receive an approximation of what you do through medical outlets?

Answer carefully.

You and future generations of chiropractors will need an answer to these questions as tremendous battles are waged in the health care

137

environment. Your motives will be tested as increasing amounts of research validates the anecdotal experiences that chiropractors have seen since 1895. As more and more within the medical community see the wisdom and cost-effectiveness of a chiropractic approach, watch, what was a vague, faceless "medical enemy" curl up and offer gifts of interest, respect, and acceptance. Just what you've always wanted. Isn't it?

This possible development could force many chiropractors to choose sides. Some will have to decide what is more important, the health of millions or the survival of chiropractic as a separate and distinct healing art. Thankfully, this decision will not likely be forced upon chiropractors in the very near future. Instead, the erosion will be subtle and conducted over the course of so many chiropractic careers, it will go largely unnoticed until the last chiropractic college closes its doors. By the time the professional journal advertising and direct mail campaigns for "Save The Fountainhead" are received, chiropractic could well be all but history.

Is chiropractic, its philosophy, its institutions, its history, and its professional membership more or less important than chiropractic results? Should chiropractic remain an "alternative" or would the highest calling be to integrate it into the mainstream?

The fact of the matter is, today, most patients who receive the benefits of chiropractic care choose not to embrace the philosophical tenets of the profession. I'm sure this is partly due to the fact that it is the rare doctor who even explains the difference between the medical perspective and the chiropractic orientation towards health, healing, and physiology. Patients may nod at the right times during new patient orientations and reports of findings, but it is rarely the sign of discarding a belief system that has served, however inade-quately, to explain germs, disease, healing, and the use of drugs and other outside-in sickness solutions.

No, chiropractic philosophy and the ramifications of its "cause" orientation is rarely discussed with patients. Patients aren't asked to reveal their understanding or assimilation of chiropractic principles. In large part, each patient's pre-consultation health attitude remains intact, during and after discontinuing care. So, while their spine may enjoy better biomechanics, their understanding and appreciation of what their chiropractor did to them is clouded by a lifetime of medical indoctrination.

If you have an interest in saving the institution of chiropractic by helping it remain distinct and separate, the following suggestions could help. If, on the other hand, you think it's about time chiropractic assimilate into the mainstream, and go the way of osteopathy, then these suggestions should be ignored.

1. Clarify your position. For a moment, raise your sights above survival, making payroll, and taking home enough money to make your car payment. How do you visualize the future for the next generation of chiropractors? What is the legacy you'll be leaving behind? How do you see it in the overall context of health care?

All too many chiropractors (and patients) have an outlook that extends only to the next paycheck, next meal, or next lottery ticket purchase. They literally can't "see" the future. Without the ability to conceive a vivid picture of the future, many become lost and disoriented. This is the source of fear and general malaise that the profession suffers from today. The future is dark, formless, and without substance. It is a widespread problem because so many lack the discipline to confront themselves and invest the time necessary to dream a big dream. Instead, countless everyday decisions are made that consciously or unconsciously attempt to protect the status quo and avoid a backwards slide. Long-range planning is perceived as a luxury when managed care is cutting your income, telling you how to part your hair, and your practice is slowly eroding.

If this profession has any hope of assuming a role of any consequence in the future of health care, it is necessary that each association, every society, and every chiropractor be able to conceive a compelling image of that future. What's yours?

2. Confront patients. No need to hit your patients over the head, but why not attempt to change their health beliefs during those occasions that they are in your office and seeking your services?

Use the moments right before you deliver your adjustments, when patients are most focused on you and what you're doing, to ask questions or make a statement. Pose hypothetical cases, situations, and problems that can serve to get the patient thinking, reveal their health attitude, and create an opportunity to share your way of looking at things. Keep it light and know when to relinquish this opportunity to a discussion of the weather and sports scores. Make sure patients will have no reason to dread your encounters or feel like they are being lectured.

Chiropractic veterans who made fine livings before the insurance era almost always share two observations. The first, that their practices were always full of entire families and the second, that most patients came in for non-back related health problems. This was accomplished largely through lectures, orientations, and clear communications. While many of today's chiropractors seem most interested in winning access to the patient's spine, 30 years ago chiropractors were interested in winning access to the patient's brain. In those days, chiropractors wanted to be an alternative to medicine.

While today the debate rages on as to whether chiropractic should be considered "alternative" or "complementary", the real issue is the perception and understanding of the patients who venture in to chiropractic offices. When I hear patients refer to their care as "chiropractic medicine" it sounds as if the marketplace has already decided our fate.

Companies like Xerox and Kleenex spend millions of dollars each year to protect their trademarked name. Xerox pleads in its advertising that Xerox is not a verb (you must not say "I xeroxed the report.") and it is not an adjective (you must not say "Please hand me the xeroxed report"). Xerox, Kimberly-Clarke, and countless other companies must defend their trademarked names, lest they loose them like the original manufacturers of bandaids, catsup, and walkmans. The same challenge faces chiropractic.

Is chiropractic, its philosophy, its institutions, its history, and its professional membership more or less important than the results it produces? If you're not sure, simply ask your next patient. ∎

PATIENT TESTING

Experts seem to agree that the educational system in our country is a disaster. It's not working. We're graduating students who can't read, write, or even think. SAT scores have plummeted, while the test scores in countless other industrialized nations seem to suggest that they are producing better students. Is it our culture? Is it the influence of television? Is it our teachers? Is it a lack of parental support and involvement? Probably.

As a high school student, I remember always wanting to know what kind of test we would be having. "Is it multiple choice, fill-in, or essay," I would ask. Thankfully, it seemed that multiple choice was a frequent testing method. Apparently it was easier for the teacher to grade. It certainly was easier to take!

Only problem is, the tests we take in real life rarely supply multiple choice answers!

The type of test most of us abhorred was the essay test. Essay tests necessitated that we had acquired some actual content and spent enough time thinking about a particular topic to form some opinions about it. Essay questions were the most difficult to answer because they required us to think and put our ideas into words.

Most patients fail when they are "tested" by essay-style questions about chiropractic, asked of them by their friends and family. "How does chiropractic work?" "I've heard that chiropractors cause strokes." "Why do you have to see a chiropractor forever?" "Why don't you go to a real doctor?" "What does your chiropractor do?"

Based upon the answers supplied by most patients, chiropractors are having the same dismal success educating their patients, as professional, full time teachers are having with their students!

This problem is more serious than simply shrugging our shoulders and blaming television. It is a symptom of the changing context in which all types of communications and specifically, teaching communications, finds itself today. Frankly, many doctors are using the equivalent of Morse Code to communicate with their patients. No wonder patients are unable to successfully explain chiropractic to others and serve as effective referral ambassadors.

Whether it's the afferent/efferent function of the nervous system, or a computer communicating with a printer, the fundamental rule on which all communication is based, is feedback. The only way the sender of a message can be sure the receiver actually received and understood the message, is to request feedback. Consider when communication accuracy is a life or death issue: air traffic control.

If you've ever monitored United Airlines Channel 9 on the audio entertainment selector, you've been able to listen in on the conversation between your pilot and the tower. It's especially interesting when landing or taking off from busy airports such as La Guardia in New York or O'Hare in Chicago. One mistake or inaccurately interpreted message could endanger the lives of hundreds of passengers. Pilots are trained to repeat back to the tower the relevant piece of information, "Copy that, 280 left" or "Descend to one-five thousand and hold," or whatever the tower has instructed the pilot to do. This completes the feedback loop and assures the sender of the message (the tower) that the receiver (the pilot) has actually received the message. But it doesn't stop there. Then, the sender of the message monitors the radar screen to confirm that the message was properly interpreted and acted upon. It's a system that works incredibly well.

In chiropractic we have the monitoring process down pat. We even have the assistance of computers to track compliance and missed appointments. But the feedback loop is clearly deficient.

During the initial stages of care, many doctors interpret a patient's total compliance as proof that the patient understood the report of findings, the implications of neglect, and has accepted the value of post-symptomatic wellness care. It's not until the patient disappears from the radar screen that many doctors are confronted with the shortcomings of their communication protocol. The most dogmatic doctors blame the patient, or the patient education video they use, or the report script supplied by their management company, or the front desk staff, or the HMO that's moved into town. It is the rare doctor who is willing to perform the self-examination necessary to question his or her communication technique.

The fact is, based on the patient communications I've observed in most offices, little feedback is demanded of the patient. Even the most ambitious doctors, who pour out their chiropractic souls at patient lectures, expect little feedback from patients other than attentive eye contact and occasional head-nodding, signaling agreement. Rarely, if ever, are patients asked to repeat in their own words, the main points of a doctor's report or lecture. So, it's no surprise that when a concerned spouse or interested co-worker asks about chiropractic, many patients are caught flat-footed, tongue-tied and take on the glassy-eyed appearance of someone who has fallen under the spell of a religious cult!

And we wonder why 100 years of great results hasn't propelled chiropractic into the forefront of the healing arts? Sadly, even patients who have had an incredibly positive chiropractic experience find it difficult to explain or defend their chiropractic encounter to someone else.

Here are two suggestions for overcoming this communication challenge:

1. Use a common language. Regardless of the native language spoken, air traffic controllers around the world speak one language: English. When huge 747s land in Hong Kong or Nairobi, the pilot and tower converse in English! Unfortunately, many chiropractors often use hard to understand dialects or an entirely different language, with esoteric idioms such as Innatese, Lesionitis, or an especially hard to understand accent called "I-don't-treat-symptomese." No wonder patients find it difficult to replicate themselves as referral ambassadors! Forget your decoder ring and chiropractic is an obscure ritual that is hard to describe and impossible to understand.

Learn ways to describe terms you take for granted, such as subluxation, adjustment, degeneration, misalignment, and other "code" words in simpler terms. Provide metaphors and pictures, or pull language from the construction trade, computer industry, telephone system, or find some other terms your patients will be able to understand and use with others who have little understanding of anatomy or physiology.

2. Ask to assure understanding. Remember, most of your patients came to your office to have their backs fixed, not to learn how to be a chiropractor! So while patient education is important, it is essential that you administer your patient education with a sense of lightness. You don't want to come off looking and sounding like a boorish professor with a one-track mind!

One way to check your patient's understanding of chiropractic is to ask a question just before you deliver your adjustment. That's when patients are most alert, expectant, and focused. Once you "give away" what they came to your office to get, your influence and their curiosity drops precipitously. It's the same reason they show the commercials and coming attractions at the movie theater *before* the main attraction. And, why they air the bulk of the TV commercials right before "who dunnit" is revealed at the end of the show. Same with your patient education. Ask your question, request feedback, uncover their understanding on each visit *before* you perform your adjustments.

While most doctors are constantly on the lookout for better ways to explain chiropractic to their patients, few are brave enough to ask the questions necessary to properly validate the success of their efforts. Yet, this is a vast, unexplored territory that offers many opportunities. The problem is *not* that your patients are dumb, or your community is more medically-oriented than the next, or that you're using the wrong patient education video. You've simply forgotten to solicit the appropriate feedback from your patients. How else can you be sure your patient education efforts are relevant or even work? ■

NEW PATIENT SONAR

As a child, and still today, I'm quite interested in submarines. I remember checking out books at the library about how submarines work. I dreamed of being a submariner. According to the books I've read, submariners were special people in the navy who could handle long periods at sea and who were short enough to easily live among the pipes, tubes, and low ceilings of a submarine. More recently, movies like *Crimson Tide* and *The Hunt For Red October* have rekindled my interest in submarines. Interestingly, playing a major role in these movies are the sonar operators who use their skills to detect and plot the movements of other ships. These men, with their highly refined skills at detecting and interpreting the sounds of different types of propellers and the echoes of sound "pings" sent out from their vessels, were doing what I always dreamed of doing.

I never became a submariner. Since I was born in 1952 I was among the very first to be exposed to the draft lottery during the Viet Nam war. On that fateful day, I had decided that if I had drawn a low number, I was going to enlist and fulfill my dream. Instead, my number was 209. They drew up to 175 that year and I ended up pursuing other dreams. I still have a high regard for the discipline and courage of those who seal themselves into submarines for months at a time to serve and protect. Today, as a communicator, I'm especially interested in the way submarines communicate and navigate the murky depths of the sunless oceans. A situation not unlike doctors who encounter a new patient.

Ping...

Sonar operators send out a sound, and the way the reflected sound returns to the submarine gives the operator an estimate of the size and distance of the object. Common boats, ships, and even whales have distinctive sonar "fingerprints." In the doctor/patient relationship, asking patients various types of questions reveals the distinctive signature of the patient's understanding, attitude, and recovery process. Not only can questions serve to reveal how close the patient is to embracing a chiropractic perspective, they can provide valuable information that can direct and personalize your patient education approaches. It is the reflected image, the responses that come back from patients that are more important than the questions themselves.

Instead of perfecting the Socratic skill of questioning, many chiropractors invest an inordinate amount of energy into learning a report of findings script, memorizing a snappy patient lecture, preforming a X-ray view box monologue, and other one-way, "data dumps" aimed at patients. The only patient feedback that registers is patient visit statistics. Ignoring the body's own afferent/efferent feedback loop, these same doctors squander valuable opportunities to enhance true patient understanding and establish the deep levels of rapport necessary in creating optimum long-term patient relationships.

Ping...

On those rare occasions when a patient asks a question, it is so easy to fall into the trap of taking a deep breath and immediately showing off what we know. Something clicks, and we play a perfectly practiced tape, revealing our training, understanding, and unique perspective. Showing off in this way is heady stuff.

What does a patient question mean? It could be an attempt at resolving some ambiguity. It could be a way of confirming a suspicion. It could be an oblique attempt at asking for help or expressing dissatisfaction. A question is not always what it seems to be. Taking patient questions entirely at face value overlooks the rich subtext of information that can dramatically shape the success of a patient relationship.

When I call the telephone directory assistance operator, I ask a question and I am given an answer. Occasionally, the operator will ask a follow-up question to clarify my request, but it will never deal with my motives, the subject matter I'm going to discuss with the person I'm calling, or even why I didn't write the number down the last time I requested it! No, it's all at face value and the interchange closely resembles the actions of a rudimentary computer.

"How long until I start feeling better?" a patient asks.

"Well, that depends..." and the doctor engages program loop #232. The question is a simple one, and most doctors, depending upon their unique outlook on chiropractic, can supply a cogent answer while simultaneously palpating the cervical spine and completing their SOAP notes. But that wasn't even the question the patient was really asking! Perhaps the patients real concern was a financial issue. Maybe a friend, upon learning that they'd begun chiropractic care, told them they'd have to go for the rest of their lives. Who knows what the hidden agenda of their questions really are?

Whether the patient asks a direct question or simply makes an observation such as, "I felt really good when I woke up this morning," ask a follow-up question that can begin to reveal the more intimate meaning of the question or observation, such as, "Why do you think that is?"

Ping...

You probably have a stock answer as to why they now feel better upon waking in the morning, but it's likely to be perceived as merely the "company line," while steamrollering over the opportunity to establish a deeper, more substantial relationship.

It's easy to imagine that patients are showing up to have their innate intelligence optimized and their human potential maximized by avoiding this type of questioning. It's easy to assume that patients want better posture or improved spinal curves because that's the recurrent theme of your adjusting room tirades. It's easy to soothe your conscience and avoid confronting a lack of referrals and continuous patient dropout by taking a deep breath and showing off how much you know. Yet, the price that is paid by not digging deeper and creating a forum for patents to divulge their real concerns or understanding is formidable.

Most doctors are good at asking questions that help reveal the patient's physical complaints. "Does that hurt here?" "Does that seem a little sore there?" "How long have you been experiencing this?" These questions, combined with various physical, orthopedic, and neurological tests can help establish an appropriate care program. However, this reduces a patient's chiropractic experience to the most superficial physical plane. Deepening the bond to include the potential for intellectual, emotional, and spiritual connections requires an exchange of better information. And that means the doctor must have enough self-confidence and presence of mind to ask questions of patients, whose answers will require more compassion, creativity, and intimacy than a well-practiced "topic of the day" monologue.

Ping...

Navigating through the medical-based health attitudes of today's patients requires every sounding device and guidance system that can be mustered. The one-size-fits-all explanations of the past barely worked then, and are especially ineffective with today's visually-oriented patients. Patients, who are uncommunicative or who are unaccustomed to confronting those in authority, can appear aloof or seem uninterested in chiropractic. Those who have a poor self-image or who feel self-conscious investing in their own health, can seem distant and unresponsive. The tragic result is countless patients who never really "connected" with their chiropractor and leave behind the storage problem of inactive files. ■

WHIPS AND CARROTS

One of the greatest challenges of any health care practitioner is to motivate patients to modify a behavior that is counter-productive to their long term health interests. Dentists beg patients to floss. Heart by-pass surgeons beg patients to stop smoking. Nutritionists beg patients to eat less fat and more fiber. And chiropractors beg patients to continue their care beyond the mere relief of obvious symptoms. Based upon the comments from these various health providers, success in changing patient behaviors is limited. Why is that?

The fact that most patients don't change their behaviors is particularly troubling to chiropractors. When patients reject what doctors see as the obvious benefits from continued chiropractic care, it seems a rejection of the doctor's highest purpose and professional calling. For health professionals who are quick to boast that they don't treat symptoms, being relatively unsuccessful at retaining nonsymptomatic patients must be a continuing source of frustration. Professional burnout is just around the corner if one's philosophy is so divergent from their real world experience. Worse, even though you may personally benefit from some type of periodic, nonsymptomatic wellness care, continued patient rejection of what seems so obvious to you, can cause you to question your career choice or even the validity of your chiropractic philosophy.

Certainly, one of the most important reasons for any type of patient education is to help patients assume the responsibility necessary to effect appropriate behavior. Yet, patient education is a broad concept. Does that mean lectures? Special visits? Videos? Group reports? Brochures? Which ones? First visit? Every visit?

If you recognize the value of wellness/maintenance/preventive care, and you're educating your patients like crazy, but not enough patients seem interested or willing to follow through with it, a change in communication tactics may be in order. Because first and foremost, there is little reinforcement in the day-to-day world of most patients to prompt non-symptomatic wellness care. In the instant gratification, if it feels good do it, win-the-lottery world most patients live in, there are few rewards or incentives for preventive, long term beneficial behaviors.

Have you been using a carrot or a whip?

It's been observed that each of us is motivated to action by either one of two reasons: to obtain a reward or to avoid a punishment. Seeking pleasure or avoiding pain are powerful inducements to get people to do anything from regularly changing the oil in their car's engine (avoiding the pain of losing money and use of their cars) to regularly mowing the lawn (the pleasure of neighbors' compliments). Do you know which motive inspires each of your patients to action?

There are several methods to uncover this motivational preference.

1. Examine their mouth. A wise chiropractor once told me that a "thorough" chiropractic examination is not complete until the patient's mouth is examined. Chances are their dental hygiene will be a good reflection of their spinal hygiene. If their mouth is a mess, they probably wait until excruciating pain prompts them to seek professional care. In the same way, that's what has prompted them to seek care in your office for their spine!

2. Determine seat belt use. Ask patients how often they use their seat belts. Always, sometimes, or rarely? Sure, in many states it's against the law not to wear them, but people's attitudes are often stronger than the fine for being caught. Not being able to visualize (and value) the possible life-threatening consequences of not wearing seat belts causes many to unnecessarily risk their lives driving to your office!

3. Eating cake. We're getting a little off the beaten path, but ask your patients anyway. In what order do they eat cake? Frosting first? Equal amounts of frosting and cake? Or do they save the frosting to the very end? Just a guess, but I bet frosting-first patients aren't likely candidates for long-term wellness care.

4. Teeth flossing. This is familiar territory, but belongs in this context, too. A patient's motive for brushing or flossing their teeth can provide some valuable insights into their likely commitment to maintaining their spine. Do they brush and floss to avoid tooth decay and gum disease, or because they want optimum health and dental hygiene? The difference is subtle, but can reveal their mindset.

Generally speaking, the majority of patients are motivated to avoid pain. Pain has prompted them to overcome the fear of the unknown and show up in your office, and when the pain goes away, they are likely to do the same. These values are formed early and are likely to remain unchanged throughout one's life. Here's the rub. Instead of whips, most chiropractors prefer the carrot approach. They seek optimal health. Many are constantly searching for the best technique, the best supplement, the best exercise program, and the best way to sustain optimal health. That's why a career in chiropractic was so appealing in the first place.

It doesn't take a vivid imagination to figure out why doctors and patients have such a hard time understanding each other. When a "whip" oriented patient finds the relief they originally sought by consulting your office, and you hold out the "carrot" of optimal health and preventing a relapse, you might as well be speaking a foreign language. No video, brochure, or lay lecture is likely to overcome their world view. Of course if a third party will pay for it and the waiting time isn't too long, even some of the most intransigent patients will avail themselves of the pampering they receive at your hands!

Does that mean you shouldn't try to inspire patients to a bigger vision of health? Try! But don't take it so personally when patients reject your overtures. Remember, their health attitudes were formed at an early age and frankly, some people actually enjoy the attention they receive when dealing with a personal health issue.

Of course the real reason to persevere is for the children of your adult patients. Regardless of their own shortcomings, most adults want the very best for their children. If future generations of chiropractors are to enjoy the fulfillment of caring for patients who want the very best for themselves, it's important that these values get communicated at an early age. Look for opportunities to introduce chiropractic to more children. Look for occasions to speak at area schools. When is career day? How can you complement the sixth grade teacher's curriculum, that right now puts such an overriding emphasis on the circulatory system instead of the nervous system? Get in front of an audience of children who aren't skeptical, who could care less about your educational achievements, and don't have the baggage about chiropractic that their parents have.

With this commitment to future generations of chiropractic patients, needless suffering can be avoided. By adjusting the attitudes and investing in the understanding of chiropractic in the youngest members of your community, you plant important seeds which someday may grow up to become carrots. ■

TALK IS CHEAP

In huge underground vaults, billions of dollars worth of diamonds, sorted by size, weight, color, and clarity, are being stored away by the DeBeers diamond cartel. By removing these diamonds from the marketplace, they have successfully controlled the availability, price, and value of "a girl's best friend." In fact, if all these diamonds were to be dumped onto the market, that expensive diamond engagement ring that took the first year of marriage to pay for, would be worth just a couple of dollars. Apparently, the universe puts little value on things which are so abundant, such as sand, opinions, and especially words. Which is why most oral efforts at educating patients produce such dismal results. Spoken words are mere pennies in the currency of communication.

A great deal of importance is placed on our ability to speak. Like learning to walk, most parents record the hour and day of their child's first utterings. The joy of this early vocabulary is quickly supplanted by the child's ability to communicate their wants and desires, and later by thoughtful, intelligent conversation. And while sociologists remind us that more than 70% of a message is communicated by our nonverbal articulations (body language, hand movement, tone, pace, facial expression, etc.), most doctors depend almost exclusively upon the words from their mouths as a means of communicating chiropractic to their patients.

There's a reason why "talk is cheap." Just about all of us are effective at arranging words into a fashion that resembles rational, thoughtful social intercourse. As others talk to us, we nod our heads and appear interested. We make and then break eye contact for the socially correct length of time and appear as if we are carefully weighing the speakers words and drinking in their meaning and implications. When, in fact, we're actually distracted by the effort of composing our response! Most "conversations" are merely two people talking *at* each other about a similar subject.

The ineffectiveness of "talking" as a communication modality is heightened in doctor/patient relationships. After the initial give and take of the consultation and information gathering phase of the relationship, the patient education and report of findings communication becomes a decidedly one-sided affair. With the exception of the sometimes subtle body language of a wary patient (potentially distorted by physical discomfort), there is little feedback that the patient is understanding, believing, or accepting the words uttered by the doctor. But this does little to slow the torrent of words flowing from the doctor's mouth. If anything, it often serves to accelerate the pace and number of words used. If patients are not bold enough or sufficiently assertive to ask for a better explanation or a needed clarification, they are simply enrolled in a care plan that seems designed to address the issue they understand perfectly—how they feel.

Unfortunately, the consequences of ineffectively talking to patients doesn't show up until several weeks or months later. This passage of time can serve to cover up a significant reason why many patients decide to discontinue care due to a lack of understanding. Like a patient in his or her 30s who is unlikely to see the relationship between their headaches and falling off their horse 20 years earlier, the lag time between the orally delivered report of findings and the resulting patient dropout covers up the connection. Instead, many doctors are misled into believing the patient understands the orally presented report because of the almost perfect compliance among patients during the earliest stages of care.

Yet, when doctors find that their well-rehearsed report or "can't fail" lecture no longer produces the results it once did, they often go out in search of a new script. New words are so inexpensive and easy to find! Seminar speakers sell them by the hour and consultants sell them by the pound. Instead of blaming the limitations of the communication channel, many search for the illusive words to charm patients into submission.

How many chiropractic seminars have you sat through? How many audio cassette programs have you listened to? How many hours of classroom lectures have you endured? How many radio newscasts have you listened to? How many sermons have you heard? More importantly, how many do you remember? The spoken word is not only hard to remember, even when delivered by an excellent speaker, but it is hard for listeners to recount what they've heard to someone else. In a chiropractic setting, this makes it difficult for patients to recreate your report of findings to a spouse who couldn't make it in, or for patients to share with others what they've learned at your new patient orientation. Depending upon the spoken word to grow your practice is like trying put out a forest fire with a squirt gun.

If chiropractic is so misunderstood and the spoken word so ineffective, how do you communicate effectively with patients? How do you give a report of findings and perform all the other communication chores necessary to inform patients, obtain their consent to begin care, and motivate them to continue?

This overdependence upon the spoken word occurred to me while I was speaking on the telephone with a doctor who has a stuttering problem. After painstakingly discussing several other topics, he asked for suggestions on how I would deal with the patient communication challenge he faces if I were him. Good question. After discarding the notion of singing his report (country singer Mel Tillis stutters when he speaks, but not when he sings) I tried to offer some practical solutions.

I suggested that he start filling the walls of his office with pictures. Pictures of Crest toothpaste users with braces, smiling from the pages of a women's magazine. Pictures from the Midas advertisement of a car receiving a front end alignment. A suit of armor. The Tin Man from the *Wizard of Oz*. And on and on. Pictures that could metaphorically demonstrate or illustrate virtually any chiropractic concept from adjustments to X-ray exposure. With an extensive library of visual resources on the walls of his clinic, all he needed to do was point to an appropriate picture and speak just a word or two. Sure, obtain the best chiropractic wall posters, and show the patient's X-rays, but create your own library of visual tools that can serve to enhance patient understanding without a long, drawn out verbal explanation.

Pictures don't have the ambiguity that the spoken word does. If you've ever tried to assemble something as simple as a bicycle on Christmas eve, or follow the directions for your new barbecue grill before your dinner guests arrive, you're already familiar with this limitation. With the exception of optical illusions, Escher prints, people with color blindness, or individuals from significantly different cultural backgrounds, pictures are pretty much the same thing for everyone. They say a picture is worth a thousand words. This chapter is about 1200 words. I could have saved you the trouble by showing you a picture of a doctor's words going in one ear and out the other while a patient is day dreaming about their vacation, followed by a picture of an adjusting room filled with pictures torn from magazines. Get the picture? ■

BUT I DON'T
TREAT SYMPTOMS

There is probably no greater form of self-deception practiced by the most philosophical chiropractors than the notion that they don't treat symptoms. When patients moan and whine about the ache or pain that prompted them to begin chiropractic care, many patients are often pushed away with a holier-than-thou, "But, I don't treat symptoms." If you could see how your patients interpret your claim, you'd be stunned.

If you consider yourself a committed chiropractor, who wants to remain true to the philosophical tenets of chiropractic, a few lessons in patient communications may be helpful. But, if your current patient orientation approach is working so well that your practice is bursting at the seams, read no further. If your established communication protocol is so successful that only similarly philosophically aligned patients of your dreams are showing up in your office, ignore the following observations.

The greatest danger a chiropractic communicator can overlook is the difference between content and context. Mix these up; ignore how they can respectively shape the perceptions of your patients, and you can end up with patients scratching their heads, feeling unwelcome in your office and afraid to share their concerns, sense of progress, or discuss other matters that affect retention and even the referral process. In other words, you can win the battle, but lose the war.

Most chiropractors have the content of their message pretty well figured out. After years of indoctrination at school and countless hours sitting on uncomfortable hotel meeting room chairs, the chiropractic message is pretty clear in their minds. Sure, some think telling the D.D. Palmer story is essential. Others believe posture or biomechanics should be the primary thrust of their patient messages. Still others reduce it down to "subluxations" and other terms patients have never heard of. Some doctors, with their eyes dilated and their mouths foaming slightly, discuss the more esoteric notions of Universal and Innate Intelligences. The beauty of chiropractic is that it seems to offer something for everyone.

Yet more dangerous and less obvious than the content of the chiropractic message is the context in which it is received, interpreted, and acted upon by patients.

Instead of the confidence that you have acquired after successfully helping hundreds of patients, patients are in fear of the unknown. Instead of the clear mind and mental faculties that you possess, their personalities and concentration are distorted by painful symptoms. Instead of dabbling in the stock market and building a portfolio of tax-free municipal bonds, patients are worried that their injury may get them fired and be unable to support their families. Instead of having a thorough understanding and appreciation of human anatomy and physiology, many patients are simply ungrateful guests in a bag of skin whose homeostatic function is largely a mystery. Instead of having a free, unlimited supply of chiropractic adjustments like you, they are victims of managed care schemes, or must increasingly pay for their care out of their own pockets.

Do you suppose the philosophical content of your message becomes just a little irrelevant in this context? More often than not, it simply confirms to them that they've consulted a whacked-out alternative care provider!

Of course the problem is, the doctor is absolutely 100% correct. Treating symptoms is the domain of medicine. In our current lexicon, "health" care is really sickness care and "health" maintenance organizations are mostly about disease treatment. When the whole notion of health is corrupted by our language and the results of a lifetime of symptom treating, your message falls on deaf ears. Flogging patients to attend spinal care classes rarely produces converts. Force-feeding videos, pamphlets, and extended reports of findings are unlikely to produce the chiropractic zealots you desire.

Find out for yourself. Ask every patient that shows up in your office tomorrow, "So, why are you here today?" Ask every patient that you indoctrinated at your last impassioned Wednesday night spinal care class, "So, why are you here today?" Ask every patient that you placed in front of a snappy patient education video, "So, why are you here today?" Ask every patient to whom you delivered a perfect report of findings, "So, why are you here today?"

If you have the courage to uncover the truth, you'll discover a gapping chasm between the warm philosophical glow you get from discussing chiropractic philosophy and the reasons your patients have for consulting your office.

Perception is everything.

Only after you are confronted by the ugly truth that patients are showing up in your office for the treatment of an obvious ache or pain will it cause you to get real. Only after you discover that your patient orientation program isn't working, will it cause you to make needed changes.

Fortunately, chiropractic is so effective, so innately correct, so deliciously simple that it works whether your patients buy your philosophical piety or not. And while the philosophy of chiropractic, with its "cause" orientation has universal applications, playing a linguistic sleight-of-hand is disingenuous.

For example, let's say your house is in serious need of some fresh paint. Unlike the philosophy you pound into your patients about prevention, health maintenance, and living a wellness life, you've waited until the need for a paint job (symptoms) is embarrassingly obvious. Even your neighbors are noticing the need for some fresh paint. "What you need is a painter," observes the neighbor across the street.

Fortunately, there's an establishment located by the big shopping mall that looks promising. Out front is a big sign, "Family Painting Center." Upon entering this little storefront you are met by a recep-tionist behind a counter. The room has a half dozen chairs, coat rack, magazines, and a brochure rack full of paint samples and color swatches.

"Good morning," you volunteer to the receptionist. "I need to get my house painted."

The receptionist looks up with an air of impatience. "What color is it now?" she asks.

"Well, it's a kind of a faded yellow color," you volunteer. "How much does it cost to have a house painted these days?"

"Well, that depends. It depends how big the house is, what type of siding you have, how many windows, how much preparation is required, and what color you want. I can't quote you a price until we actually see your house," she says with an expression bordering on disdain.

Sensing that this painting contractor doesn't want your business, you decide to persevere with caution. "Do you folks use brushes and rollers or do you spray the paint on?"

"I think you'd better have a seat. I'll get the color specialist and he can answer your questions," she says with a heavy sigh.

After disappearing briefly, she returns to escort you to a small consultation room. "Someone will be with you in just a moment."

Surveying the room you see whole rainbows of paint chips. One entire wall is a display showing the history of the paint brush. To another wall several posters are mounted, showing various homes before painting and after painting. Suddenly the door opens and a man in his middle 40s enters the room. He is dressed in white overalls that, while nicely pressed, are covered with a constellation of paint splatters.

"Hi, my name is Doc," he says extending his right hand and turning it into a firm, two-handed handshake. "How can I help you?"

"Well, as I was explaining to the woman out front, I need to have my house painted."

"I'm sure she told you that we don't paint houses," he says with a perfectly serious expression.

"I don't understand, I thought..."

"We colorize houses. We change them from one color to another," he says brightly.

"You use paint?"

"After preparing the surface, we use colorizing agents that modify the reflective properties of the particular home," he says without breaking a smile.

"About these colorizing agents. How are they applied to my house?" you ask, with similar seriousness.

"That varies. Each house is treated individually. With some we use brushes, on others we use rollers, and still others we spray the colorizing agent onto the surface. First we conduct a thorough examination of your house and then we suggest some colors."

"How much do you generally charge?"

"Again, that depends. Do you have color insurance or are you a member of a color maintenance organization?"

"Why should that matter?" you ask as your frustration begins to show. "I just want my house painted!"

"Now please remember, we don't paint houses. We colorize them."

Stunned, you pause for a moment and collect your thoughts. "Hold on now. Let me get this straight. You don't paint houses?"

"No, we colorize them."

"Okay, you colorize them. You'll change the color of my house by applying paint over..."

"Applying a colorizing agent," he says quickly correcting you.

"Okay, you apply a colorizing agent over the old paint, and my house will look better," you say, summing up your understanding of the services this fellow renders. "That's what I really want. I want my house to look better."

"I can't guarantee it'll look better. All I do is change the color. If by chance it doesn't look better, I won't take the blame. But then on the other hand, if afterwards it looks great, I won't take the credit either. My job is to simply colorize the exterior. Is that what you want?" he asks with an I-don't-really-need-your-business attitude.

He looks honest. He sounds qualified. His before and after

pictures of other homes seem impressive. But there's something just a little kooky about this guy...

The fact is, subluxations are symptoms. If you really want to concern yourself with cause, join the thought police and make sure your patients avoid stress, negative thoughts, and emotional upsets. If you really want to avoid treating symptoms, crusade against learning how to walk, climbing trees, riding horseback, being a passenger in an automobile, and the other causes of subluxations. Better yet, rally against being born in the first place—the birth process may be the most traumatic thing we endure!

During the early stages of chiropractic care after your new patient orientation and indoctrination, it's easy to interpret loyal compliance as a sign that you've made a difference in a patient's understanding of true health.

But you haven't.

While still basking in the affirmation from conducting your 100th spinal care class, it's tempting to think that patients are racing home to flush their inventory of lotions, potions, and pills down the toilet.

But they're not.

In the course of discouraging patients from discussing their symptoms or volunteering their subjective improvement, it's easy to create a something that looks like patient understanding.

But it isn't. ■

PHILOSOPHICAL CAMOUFLAGE

Perhaps one of the most difficult concepts to communicate at seminars and speaking engagements is the idea that compliance or referrals or even so-called "success" is the result of what you *are*, not what you *do*. I can tell this confounds the most analytical in the audience because they ask questions that seem like requests for a recipe or a four-step process or an instruction book-like answer. Isn't it ironic that there are practices that would be the envy of just about any doctor, that use adjusting techniques you think are bogus, patient protocols you think invite malpractice, and patient financial policies you think are scurrilous?

Remember, it's not what you do, it's what you *are*.

It starts in school. Apparently, each student must choose his or her primary adjusting technique. Various adjusting "club" bulletin boards shout from the hallways like the sirens in the Odyssey, tempting students to the hidden reefs of dogma. Each claims to be the best "this" or offer the better "that." Students must get the incorrect impression that they must choose the correct adjusting technique to best assure their chances at making the money and attaining the prestige they secretly seek. Nothing could be further from the truth. It's not "what" adjusting technique you use, it's how well you use it.

Then, issues of procedure rear their ugly heads. Adjust on the first visit or the second? Lab jackets or shirt and tie? X-rays or no X-rays? What's the best way to hire staff? What are the best hours to practice? The questions and protocol choices create a vortex of doubt which ultimately sabotages the confidence and passion that a patient seeks in a doctor. Again, it doesn't matter. And while this makes neophytes uncomfortable, like technique, the issue is one of competence. If you "own" the rationale, if you've studied the pros and cons, if you have total confidence in your choice—so will your patients. But drop a beat, seem unclear, offer too many choices, appear tentative for even a split second when confronted with a question or comment, and you'll be found out! They'll chew you up and spit you out!

"Why reinvent the wheel?" goes the thinking. But, looking over your shoulder to see what someone else did or does, usurps your power and turns you into an impotent automaton. Like the Hollywood backlots, with their false-front western main streets and "New York" streetscapes, taking the shortcut of adopting someone else's procedures, creates a facade that patients can see through. A patient question, comment, or simply an unwillingness to go along with your borrowed "policy," can reveal your (or a staff member's) lack of depth, understanding, and commitment. The red flag goes up and patients naturally flee.

There are no shortcuts. Cutting in front of the line, lying, cheating, "getting an old test," or mindlessly incorporating the procedures of some other "successful" doctor may seem like you're making progress, but in reality you're merely treading water. You're simply prolonging the lessons to be learned at the School of Hard Knocks. The counterfeiter is always caught, and the knock-off is never as desirable as the real thing.

It all starts with your belief system. While there are a few rare individuals with Herculean self-control or yoga-like concentration who can fool a lie detector test, most of us give non-verbal clues when there is an inconsistency or incongruency between what we've done and what we believe. While we may not be consciously aware of a change in someone else's breathing, blood pressure, galvanic skin response, or eye dilation, researchers suggest that the primitive area of our brains can detect and evaluate these subtle clues in others. Doctors who use someone else's procedures, patient scripts, or practice policies, must think they can somehow overcome their sabotaging body language that results from adopting a behavior or script that is disconnected from the philosophy that germinated it. Nice try.

The fact is, it's the rare individual, doctor or patient, who takes the time or has the discipline to inspect his or her belief system sufficiently to reach conclusions about anything. Instead, we look to our media personalities, television, trend setters, and others equally unqualified for guidance in what we should eat, what we should wear, what we should think, and what we should believe. How else can you explain the oat bran phenomenon, high heeled shoes, evening television "news" programs, and the widespread belief that Elvis faked his own death?

If you take an inventory of the chiropractic profession's most influential leaders, there is a consistent common denominator. Even those who suggest ideas and procedures in 180 degree opposition share this commonality. They, unlike many of their followers, have taken the time to reach certain conclusions about the world, and have drawn up a philosophical underpinning that helps them either control, explain, or predict outcomes to their actions and the actions of others. Having this philosophy encoded in every fiber of their bodies is the only way to successfully project the confidence and credibility necessary to motivate an audience or exhibit the passion needed for real leadership. It is the subtle, missing ingredient in practices that have adopted the procedures, policies, and reports of someone else.

Whether you're trying to lead a group of chiropractors or shepherd a group of patients, investing the effort to identify key chiropractic issues and reaching your own conclusions about them will enhance your practice. Quick! Give an organized 30-second talk (in patient understandable language) on the following topics: Immunizations. Antibiotics. First visit adjusting. Patient education. Recalls. Paperwork. The necessity of X-rays. Managed care. Reception room reading material. Financial policy. Hours. Staff meetings. Adjusting room conversations. Staff dress code. Travel cards. The list is endless. Add to this list the 20 most commonly asked patient questions and you have a lot of thinking to do. Better yet. Put each topic or question on a 3" X 5" index card. Mix them up and have your spouse or staff test your responses. Monitor your use of language, metaphors, word pictures, and other communication enhancing devices.

The fact is, you already have a practice philosophy. Perhaps it's a patchwork derived from a career of seminars, a plaid affair from mixing and matching, or jungle camouflage that is hard to see and helps you fit in and be liked by patients. Some of it is based on false assumptions or is based on ideas that simply no longer serve you, but you've got a philosophy. Your mission is to learn ways of exhibiting it for the benefit of your patients and staff. Again, there are no shortcuts. Like the first time you tried to adjust a patient, cut yourself some slack and give yourself some time to become skillful and resourceful in the articulation of your ideas and point of view. Because while the simplicity and effectiveness of chiropractic can be quite attractive to patients, it's not what you do, it's who you are! ■

BELIEF BEFORE ACTION

I'm still astonished by the countless established doctors with years of experience under their belts, who sign up for practice management programs. After spending thousands of dollars each year (and that's just for the air fares, meals, hotels, and lost work time!) they report little statistical or emotional improvement, yet they are often talked into signing up again, because they are told, "even the best singers have singing coaches and the best ballplayers have batting coaches."

Worse than laying out all the time and money, the keys to practice success are handed out on a silver platter and many doctors simply turn up their noses like children, unhappy with the vegetable du jour.

After attending the free introductory seminar, and carefully sizing up a few competing firms, doctors sign up and then pick and choose what they will implement! Isn't this the philosophy that got medicine into trouble, thinking of the body as merely a collection of independent parts that can be isolated, studied, and controlled? Some choose to keep a new patient procedure from their previous management company, a staff hiring procedure learned from a friend across town, a report of findings approach they learned while in school, and a patient recall program taught by a charismatic doctor who had a huge practice in 1979. It doesn't take a rocket scientist to predict that this patchwork of procedures, based upon differing values, personalities, and practice objectives, is bound for failure. Seems to me that if you hire a coach, you should do *everything* he or she tells you. Everything.

"But Bill, I gotta be me!"

Yes, it *is* a profession of Lone Rangers. Doctors want "success," only if it can be on their own terms.

The dirty little secret about practice management is that there are no secret handshakes, scripts, or brass lamp rubbing procedures, that when implemented, result in "through the roof" success for every doctor. There are no shortcuts, no magic pills, and no sure-fire-this-will-work-every-time procedure. Oh sure, there are always a few juicy testimonials spouting lurid statistics that seem to validate this month's gimmick, but of course, "your mileage may vary." Doctors who don't get the same results as the charming namesake of the management organization are then blamed as having deficient self-esteem, confrontational skills, or a poverty complex. It's the perfect scam.

What few seem to recognize is that virtually all behaviors are the result of one's governing belief system. If you believe post X-ray changes aren't really possible, guess what happens? If you believe staff members are basically lazy and dishonest, guess what happens? If you're convinced the only way to survive in the 1990s is to depend upon third parties, guess what?

If you don't hold the same belief system as the person revealing how they made a million dollars, guess what happens when you get home and try to reproduce their recipe with your patients?

If you're going to be successful acquiring a new skill, implementing a new procedure, or breaking an old habit, it's helpful to first model your teacher or mentor's belief system. While it's tempting to take notes, trying to record the step-by-step process, hoping to avoid an implementation mistake, the place you should start is with the underlying philosophy, value system, and track record of the person making the suggestion! Walt Disney World exists and has filled millions of families with joy because of the beliefs of Walt Disney, not because of the park location, admittance fees, or that the park is encircled by a narrow gauge railroad. Wal-Mart exists because of the vision and beliefs of Sam Walton, not because of the greeter, the shelving system, or type of high pressure sodium lights used to illuminate the stores. The tangible parts of these respective kingdoms, the procedures, scripting, concrete, steel, and glass are merely manifestations of a belief system. The decision to use one material or procedure over another is an extension of the point of view and philosophy being operated upon. Procedures and scripts almost invent themselves when everyone involved is grounded in the purpose and long term objectives of the endeavor.

What are the beliefs guiding the decisions made in your practice? Are your procedures and patient protocols congruent with your beliefs?

Honest/dishonest. Do you believe people are basically honest or dishonest? Moreover, if you encounter a dishonest person, are you likely to be a sufficient influence to make them honest? What you believe, reflects in your behavior, your procedures, and everything about your practice. It's been my experience that only a small fraction of people are dishonest. If I'm only moderately alert I can generally avoid encounters with them. Becoming one of the targets of those I am unable to recognize, I try to forgive, and try even harder not to change my core belief. Remember, "people rarely steal because they are poor. They are poor because they steal."

Benevolent/Malevolent. Do you believe the world you live in is basically safe, or is it a fearful place? Again, the undertones of your choice (and it is a choice) are exhibited in countless behaviors—everything from your office location, layout, and security system, to your willingness to refer to other chiropractors or your attitude about medical doctors. Probably the one thing that affects this crucial belief in all too many people in our culture is television. Based upon the newscasts and "entertainment" programming choices of many stations, you might start thinking murderers are lying in wait in every mall parking lot and random acts of violence could occur at just any moment. I don't believe it.

Money as purpose or byproduct. This is a revealing belief. Those who wait to win the lottery often subscribe to the notion that they will be _____ (fill in the blank with happy, fulfilled, sexy, successful, liked, etc.) when they finally win the lottery. As if the lack of money is the cause of their predicament! Just about every financial problem is a spending problem, not an earning problem. And the universe will reward you only to the degree that you add value to others. The more value you add, the more you make. What adds more value? The temporary relief of headaches and low back pain or keeping a patient well so they can enjoy life to the fullest? Treating symptoms after they appear or caring for children to prevent problems from developing? Your income is a symptom. Find it's cause.

Abundance/scarcity. During the Jimmy Carter era, the doom-sayers were predicting that in the very near future we would be running out of petroleum for the production of gasoline, plastics, and other products. What they overlooked was something called fuel injection. Thanks to this microchip technology that can more efficiently deliver fuel to today's automobile engines, our supply of crude oil literally doubled without even discovering more reserves in the ground! We don't live in a zero-sum world where my gain automatically results in your loss. What accounts for countless chiropractic offices reporting their biggest years yet, while others are bemoaning the fact that they're 30% down over last year? It has nothing to do with location, the economy, third parties, or traffic counts in front of your office.

Long term/short term. Are you a new patient hunter and gatherer or a new patient farmer? Hunters and gatherers are always looking for the easy pickings at eye level. Once an area is adequately gleaned of the most accessible patients, they move on, looking for another overlooked or undeveloped crop. On the other hand, doctors who farm for patients are much more aware of the local ecology. They dig deep roots in the communities they've chosen to live and practice in. They make decisions and treat patient relationships in ways that will most likely foster respect for themselves, their children, and their children's children. In fact, every idea, every word spoken, and every action taken is made with one eye on the present and both eyes on the eternal future.

Inside out/outside in. In the context of a chiropractic practice this is one of the most telling beliefs! Do you believe real solutions come from the outside-in or are administered from the inside out? If you're clear on the universality of this belief, the next step is to consistently apply it! If you believe the most elegant and effective solutions come from the inside out, you naturally believe that the lack of new patients is the result of a subluxation inside your office. You name it, patient compliance, retention, collections, referrals; they are merely symptoms. The cause (that you can do anything about) is most likely to be found somewhere inside your practice. Outside-in solutions such as advertising, intimidating policies, abusive recall programs, and even asking for referrals may offer temporary relief, but they only treat the most obvious and superficial problems.

When we believe one thing but do another, we are living a lie. No one wants to invest his or her spirit in a compromise—neither doctors, staff members, or patients. When we take the wide, well-worn path of least resistance we do ourselves a great disservice. Not only are the lies we tell ourselves the most destructive emotionally, they are the ones that we spend so much time and energy protecting from discovery by others. Worse, we think we are actually being successful at hiding them! ∎

WHY ASK WHY?

Anyone who has spent time around small children has witnessed techniques that would cause the boldest investigative reporter to blush from embarrassment. "Why's that man in a wheelchair?" "Why is the sky blue?" "Why are oranges called oranges?" "Why do dogs have four legs and we only have two?" "Why?" It's a four year-old's favorite question. It is a question that most of us outgrow as we form opinions and accept reality as immutable. It's funny that while chiropractors are quick to ask "why" when diagnosing a patient's health problem, asking it to uncover the cause of a lack of new patients, staff turnover, patient dropout, and dozens of other practice-related problems is often avoided. Asking "why?" more frequently could help solve a lot of problems.

Having studied the creative process and participated in countless "brainstorming" sessions, I am always surprised at the alarming number of people who don't consider themselves "creative." While I think this can become a self-fulfilling prophecy, the fact is, each of us is immensely creative. How else can you explain our success with the rationalizations we make to justify our success-sabotaging personal behaviors? You don't think you're creative? How come you think you need a new car? Not creative? How come you haven't fired the staff person applying the brakes to your practice at the front desk? Not a creative bone in your body? How come you didn't refer that problem patient to a chiropractor who uses an entirely different technique?

Based upon the justifications that we often use to justify our behaviors, we can become unbelievably creative, when we need to.

Asking "why?" can help get to the underlying cause of a problem. Does the following conversation remind you of the concentric layers of an onion?

"On what patient visit do you generally render your first chiropractic adjustment?"

"Typically, on the first visit."

"Why?"

"I think patients have come to the office expecting me to render some type of care to help them."

"Why?"

"Oh, probably because they've gotten used to receiving some type of first-visit treatment from medical doctors."

"Why?

(The time between the question and the answer is starting to lengthen.) "Well, probably because the medical approach allows for first visit recommendations."

"Why?"

"I guess because most medical doctors only prescribe from a relatively narrow spectrum of drugs."

"Why?"

"I don't know."

"Okay, so tell me, why do you adjust on the first visit?" "Uh... I don't know."

My point isn't about the pros and cons of adjusting on the first visit, it's about our relentless pursuit and defense of the status quo. Most doctors have adopted procedures, implemented patient protocols, and have tried to adhere to policies that have not been put to the "why?" test since their inception, sometimes years ago. The result? Offices that are dangerously out of step with today's changing practice environment. If you had the good fortune to practice during the insurance era, and haven't taken the time to rethink every policy, every procedure, and every other detail about your practice, this is your wake-up call. Unfortunately, as many doctors see their practices slowly vanish, their only "why?" question is, "Why me?"

Since beginning chiropractic care on a nonsymptomatic basis in 1981, I have found that the most valuable aspect of chiropractic has been its philosophical tenets. The simplicity of looking for the "cause" instead of treating symptoms, is one of the most profoundly helpful ideas I have ever known. Recognizing this principle, and regularly practicing it, gives just about anyone in the pursuit of just about anything, an almost unfair advantage. Certainly the very survivability of chiropractic these last 100 years is a witness to the invincible power of looking to cause!

For a profession based on the notion of looking to the cause of a patient's health problem, when it comes to the health of a practice, a lack of new patients, high staff turnover, or any other challenge, there's a whole lot of symptom treating. It's as if chiropractic philosophy is only useful when there is a spine-related problem! But the philosophy of "cause" is universal. Its value and solution-producing insights can be applied to just about everything from child-rearing to vacation planning. If you just keep asking "why?" long and often enough, you can peel back enough layers of symptom treating and this-is-the-way-we've-always-done-it status quo, that can help produce fresh solutions.

Ask yourself "why?" and peel a few of the following onions and prepare yourself for some practice breakthroughs:
- Not quoting fees over the telephone
- Joining an HMO
- Hiring staff members who refuse chiropractic care
- Not holding regular and frequent staff meetings
- Not calling the patient after the first adjustment
- Yellow page advertising
- Making routine visit appointments
- Not conducting regular progress examinations
- Suing patients
- Scolding a patient for poor compliance
- Adopting the same office hours as every other chiropractor

Granted, it's hard work to take the time and energy required to question some of these fundamental beliefs or practice protocols. Yet, doing so is an essential ingredient for having a practice that remains relevant to patient needs and is skillful at adapting to a continuously changing environment. It's ironic that doctors adroit at detecting the lack of proper movement in a patient's spine, are so inclined to sanction fixations in their practices, office environments, procedures, and patient relationships.

Maybe taking the time to continually rethink the practice is a luxury. Maybe too many people subscribe to the old adage, "If it ain't broken, don't fix it." And maybe in the process they overlook ways to progressively improve their practices. Sometimes it takes the resignation of an experienced and seemingly irreplaceable staff member. Sometimes it is the breakup of a marriage. Or an automobile accident. Or a sudden drop in your take-home pay. Or burnout. Instead, like the tectonic plates along a fault line, pressure builds up until finally there is an earthquake—revolution instead of evolution. Unpleasant as these situations are, this "slipping and checking" is often the way in which our lives are "adjusted" and we are able to jump the ruts of habit, convenience, or simply the tyranny of the status quo and assume a more fulfilling life.

Some will debate whether we are such creatures of habit that meaningful change is only made at the barrel of a gun. And for others, change can be so disorienting that we want to elude its grasp at all costs. For many of us, that cost is the very life we're trying protect. Why? ■

AN ACCIDENT
WAITING TO HAPPEN

I grew up in one of those strict, children-are-to-be-seen-and-not-heard families. I'm glad I did. My brother and I were trained to say "please" and "thank you." And to write personal thank yous after receiving birthday and Christmas gifts. We were taught to turn the water faucet off tightly to avoid drips, to turn the lights out if we weren't using them, and to quickly close the refrigerator door so as not to allow too much expensive cold air to escape. The sensitivities to these concerns have continued to serve me in my later years, much to the chagrin of my own family. But, there is one lesson I learned that has served me more than the rest.

When confronted by some shortcoming, missed mark, or un-reached expectation, my brother and I would simply mumble that "It was an accident." We would be quickly corrected.

"There's no such thing as an accident," dad would say, "Every-thing has a cause."

Wow! Just think of the possibilities when you grow up learning that everything has a cause. Can you think of a better gift you could give a child?

Recognizing that everything has a cause is something that few people learn until later in life, and sometimes not even then. I meet countless people bumbling from one disaster to the next—oblivious that they are often the cause of their own misfortunes. Like a pinball, bouncing from cushion to cushion, these individuals have become victims, at the mercy of gravity, opinions, and circumstances seem-ingly out of their control.

I believe it was Albert Einstein who postulated that a problem cannot be solved from within the problem, but must come from a superior level. The only way to truly see the forest is to get up above and look down, otherwise your view is obstructed by the very trees you're trying to see! If you lack the objectivity, or the skills necessary to quiet the fears clouding your objectivity, then one feels supremely trapped. "Damned if I do, damned if I don't."

Ever build a house out of a deck of playing cards? Without a good foundation, it is impossible to build one very high. A shaky foundation makes it difficult to exceed more than two or three levels. While it appears that your house of cards collapsed because of that final card, the real problem was a poor foundation. Symptoms are like that. Whether its the symptoms surrounding a patient's lack of health, or the symptoms of a lack of new patients. The most convenient suspect is the outermost layer of the onion.

Using inductive reasoning, an observer from a alien planet might surmise that a yellow traffic light means speed up! We often use this same style of logic to explain everything from staff turnover to a patient's disinterest in learning about chiropractic. While convenient, this form of outside-in reasoning rarely provides the foundation necessary to draw accurate solutions that stand up to real world tests. Instead, symptoms are treated with vengeance, only to discover still newer symptoms emerge. Chasing symptoms is the full time occupation of many in our culture who lack the perspective, insight, or courage to face the underlying causes of their problems.

Getting to the cause of a problem is not new for chiropractors. Many proudly proclaim to patients that, "I don't treat the symptoms of your problem, I'll locate and help correct the cause." With their puffed out chests and the patient acknowledging that that makes perfect sense, they begin the examination and care routines that have given chiropractic such an enviable success record. Too bad this same philosophy isn't applied to the many challenges these same doctors face in their offices!

Lack of new patients. This is a symptom. It's cause? It could be a million and one things. Instead of trying to identify its cause, all too many chiropractors look for a gimmick (let's do a patient appreciation day), or address the symptom directly (let's do a mall show), or throw money at the symptom (let's add red ink to the yellow page ad). There is a cause for the lack of new patients, and it has nothing to do with advertising, giving away free services, or chasing prospective patients down the mall with a plastic spine. As all too many chiropractors observe to their headache patients that they don't have a lack of aspirin, offices that lack new patients don't have a lack of location, advertising, or promotions. How do you explain the offices with poor locations, no advertising, and no promotions that get plenty of new patients?

Lots of new patients. The reverse is true, too. Lots of new patients is a symptom. While those suffering from this wonderful symptom rarely investigate its cause, it is a symptom nonetheless. Interestingly, having a lot of new patients can be the cause of other symptoms, such as poor retention. The point is symptoms are not intrinsically good or bad, they just are. How one *interprets* symptoms is the critical issue. This is the flaw among some of the most philosophical chiropractors who have a mistaken notion that they shouldn't talk about the patient's symptoms lest patients place too much value on them. Sorry, but by the time most patients show up in a chiropractic office, a lifetime of medical symptom treating will not be swayed by shunning the subject! Instead, help patients interpret their symptoms (or lack of symptoms) more appropriately.

Staff turnover. Here's a serious symptom that quietly undermines patient confidence. Few patients will wonder aloud why the doctor can't seem to keep staff from leaving, yet it suggests to patients that the doctor has some shortcomings that blemish the high esteem they want in a doctor. Again, there can be many causes, and if the doctor attempts to address the wrong one, he or she can be misled into thinking the advertisement was faulty, the interview process was mishandled, or the training process deficient. While all are possible causes, what about poor doctor/staff communications? What about unmet promises made by the doctor? What about a lack of trust, creating a self-fulfilling prophecy? What about a lack of acknowledgement, praise, and encouragement? What about the doctor's expectation that the staff have mind-reading skills? Like the most difficult and complicated practice problems, it's not enough to address a cause, it must be the *real* cause.

Patients refuse patient education. Another symptom is patients who don't want to watch a video, attend a spinal care class, or devour the educational tracts in the brochure rack. The easiest culprit to blame is the video (must be too long) or time-tested lecture (it's always worked in the past) or the patient brochures (wrong brand). The real cause can be anything from not explaining the patient benefits of the educational materials (get well faster, save money, avoid a relapse) to not setting proper patient expectations ("Plan to spend about an hour with us on your first visit.") to a staff member who fails to recognize the importance of patient education, to other even more subtle causes. Symptom treating, such as making the lecture or video mandatory, or better yet, discontinuing your patient education efforts all together, becomes the cause of other even more distasteful symptoms!

Like determining the cause of a patient's health complaint, one must accept the afferent/efferent communication pathways of the nervous system as a physiological reality. Same with the other challenges in the office. Without proper feedback loops between doctor, staff, and patients, locating the cause of the problem is virtually impossible. When these relationships experience trauma, are under tension, or are toxic to any one of the parties, the truth becomes hidden.

Many doctors will pay consultants thousands of dollars for advice the staff would freely volunteer, if they weren't in fear of losing their jobs. Patients would explain countless ways the doctor could expand and grow the practice, if they thought the doctor would actually listen. Unsure, lost, and feeling isolated, many doctors find their practices and their belief structures fixated on the past. Deciding to delay or postpone a decision is like the poster in your examination room aimed at patients, "The six most dangerous words: I Thought It Would Go Away."

Success and personal fulfillment in a wide variety of disciplines isn't any more complicated than this: find the cause, address the cause, and eliminate the cause. Symptom treating may be accepted, it may be politically correct, and it usually offers the least resistance. But treating symptoms doesn't work. Never has worked. Never will work. On those few occasions when treating symptoms seemed to work, it was probably just by accident! ■

DESIGNER JEANS
FOR THE BLIND

At a time when there have been strident arguments for and against the North American Free Trade Agreement and international entanglements of the General Agreement of Tariffs and Trade, it has become more and more difficult to categorize what country produces a product. Computers are routinely designed in the U.S., their microchips and display screens are constructed in Japan, and they are often assembled in Mexico. What country "made" it? Another example is a joint venture between Mitsubishi of Japan and General Motors in the U.S. This partnership produced a car that was marketed by both companies. While virtually identical cars ("Talon" by General Motors and the "Eclipse" by Mitsubishi) the Japanese labeled Eclipse outsold the Talon by a significant margin. The only difference between the two automobiles was the name riveted to the body. This is why chiropractic research is so important. Verifying chiropractic, by having those who are supposedly "objective," with letters after their names, can be a powerful testimonial. It can influence buying decisions.

Looking to others for approval and verification is well entrenched by the onset of puberty. This is when we choose the social group we will belong to, what values and ethics we will live by, what image we will project, and what we will believe. During times of confusion it is tempting to look to others for direction. During times of change it is comforting to embrace the beliefs of those who seem more powerful, attractive, or who project confidence. Witness the recent defection of thousands of chiropractors to the whims of managed care organizations. Watch the glazed expressions of those hypnotized by television, or vicariously living their lives through the exploits of a sports team. Instead of the rugged individualism that made our nation great, most of us are getting subluxations by constantly looking over our shoulders for direction from our neighbors, work associates, or peer group. We have become sheep, who are more interested in being politically correct, than to expend the effort to produce (and defend) an original thought or idea.

The chiropractic profession could probably benefit from the "vouching" by others that is offered by more research. But the call for more research money for low back pain studies is a needless waste of resources. The efficacy and cost-effectiveness of chiropractic (and/or "spinal manipulation" in the vernacular of the research community) is already well established. If you're still in doubt, consult the findings of the RAND Organization, the State of Virginia Assessment, the Manga Report, and 35 other studies conducted in the U.S. since 1945. Instead, the research that's really needed is on the value of chiropractic care for systemic problems, organic disorders, and aging.

Why do we need more research? Two reasons.

1. To prove to the world that chiropractic works. Since the beginning of the Industrial Age, when we sent out scientists to measure, explain, and tame the world, we have become infatuated with science. It became unfashionable to "believe" in the myths of the past. Patent medicines of the late 1800s were "scientifically" formulated. Businesses applied the "scientific method" to everything from improving assembly line production, to researching the desires of customers. Phrases like "control groups" and "placebo" became part of our everyday language. Science became king. If you couldn't use one or more of your five senses to observe, measure, or document some aspect of reality, then it was not to be believed. "I'll believe it when I see it," became the watchword.

Then, along comes Einstein and the general theory of relativity, suggesting a relationship between energy and matter. Later, nuclear physics and quantum mechanics become accepted by the mainstream research community. Increasingly more and more of what researchers were discovering about the world had to be observed indirectly on photographic plates or computer modeling. Perhaps more significantly, researchers began to discover they could affect the outcome of experiments by their thoughts, expectations, and even prayers! Suddenly, reality took on a new dimension.

While much of the research community has embraced this vitalistic world view, the general public remains fixated on a mechanistic, Newtonian notion of health and human physiology. Most people see their bodies as machines (a la *The Six Million Dollar Man*), that take in resources (food, water, air, etc.) and turn them into energy. The special functionality of organs are considered separate (like capacitors, resistors, and transformers of an electronic circuit) and their interrelationships with other body parts are ignored.

Most patients enter a chiropractic office with this notion of their bodies. Sadly, most patients *leave* a chiropractic office with this notion intact. They begin care thinking they have a "low back" problem, and leave thinking their low back problem has been cleared up. And no wonder. In most chiropractic offices patients are assaulted with models of bones, X-rays of bones, and adjustments to move bones. In most chiropractic offices there is more attention given to bones than nerves and what the nerves do. Perhaps this explains why there is such interest in doing still more research on back pain and documenting the effects of whiplash.

Chiropractic research that ferrets out still more "authorities" to vouch for chiropractic can have a positive affect on the profession. Yet, unfortunately, too many doctors within chiropractic are crying for more research for an entirely different reason; to convince themselves.

2. To prove chiropractic works to chiropractors. Review the research studies being conducted by chiropractors and a whole different picture emerges. Read the reports of research monies being handed out and it sounds like those doing the research simply need assurance that what they do even works. Meanwhile, their less analytical peers are busy helping patients! What often makes their insecurities even more apparent is their methods. The conventional research community often chides chiropractic researchers for their sloppy techniques and reporting styles. Because too many chiropractors have a point to prove, and their "scientific" methods are less than untarnished, chiropractic research by chiropractors becomes suspect.

Ironically, if you're one of those chiropractors who has doubts about the validity of your career choice, seeking additional experts to prove chiropractic has value, is viable, or even works, is futile. Seeking validation from others is essentially a fear-based response to life. The apparent mistrust of your own judgment, sabotages your ability to make a difference. Becoming externally focused on the opinions of others, sets us up for disappointment. How much validation is enough? Like other fear-based responses to life (seeking power, control, security, money, etc.), you can never get enough of it. (I'm reminded of a doctor in the Seattle area who had accumulated a million dollars in tax-free municipal bonds and was working on his second million.) When is enough, enough?

Doctors who are making the greatest impact in their communities and having the most fun, don't need any more validation than the experience they receive every day in their own practices. They don't need the name of a famous designer sewn on their shirts to feel real. And they don't fall for the latest fad or embrace trendy political correctness. They are too busy loving, serving, and changing the world to care. What's your excuse? ■

ON COMMON GROUND

There is an interesting chiropractic subgroup on the Internet called chirolist (see page 229). This newsgroup offers the opportunity for computer literate chiropractors to come together to discuss various chiropractic issues. This forum is conducted by the exchange of brief e-mail messages which are distributed automatically to subscribers to the list. You'd think it would be the perfect forum to uncover the truth, assist fellow chiropractors, and exchange valuable information. Well, sometimes.

The same territorial mentality that produces nations, flags, and emigration laws on planet earth, has been extended into cyberspace. It's no surprise that one of the first tasks performed by Neil Armstrong on the moon was to plant a U.S. flag on the Sea of Tranquility. This same territorial motive has extended itself into cyberspace as contributing chiropractors choose up sides between the philosophical-whole-body-subluxation faction and the scientific-research-neuromuscular-skeletal faction. Neither party seems capable of a healthy debate that doesn't eventually degenerate into personal attacks and name calling.

It occurs to me that if this schism is not adequately resolved, the vibration and harmonics of this argument will eventually tear apart the profession. Both parties have the potential of being correct as the last rites are being administered to this honorable, if not misunderstood profession!

Can we at least agree that regardless of the philosophical bent of the practitioner, or the number of initials after the doctor's name, that

187

chiropractic care appears to have a relatively high success rate in helping patients? Can we at least agree that chiropractors do something that produces an unusually high level of patient satisfaction?

It's ironic that at about the same time the upper echelons of research in quantum mechanics and high energy physics are talking about the impact of prayer and how the thoughts of the researchers affect the outcome of their experiments, many chiropractors are prepared to write off the vitalistic aspects of chiropractic care as being "unscientific" or lacking sufficient validating research. As the scientific community is prepared to embrace the ambiguity produced by experiments whose outcomes are affected by mental energy, some chiropractors, bent on being "accepted," "valid" and "real" have fallen hopelessly in love with scientism.

For those who need research, there will never be enough. Those who have never seen a miracle, probably won't. Ever. Those who need outside authority to bolster their decisions, will go wanting.

Those who need to understand the "mechanism" or rationale of a treatment protocol before delivering it, should probably also avoid driving a car with an automatic transmission or anti-lock brakes. Patients are not mechanisms! In the same way that chiropractic worked before you knew how to adjust the spine, chiropractic can have positive affects in non-spinal health problems without knowing why or how. Or, even being repeatable. Or, without double blind clinical studies.

Certainly that's the trap in the medical domain. Give a particular set of symptoms a name, and then by definition, treatment protocol outcomes should be measurable. But in chiropractic, in which the doctor is merely helping to normalize the function and inborn healing ability of the patient, predicting an outcome, such as treating stomach pain, is virtually impossible. The doctor's intent is almost irrelevant. Only the body has the power to do something for that stomach. For all the doctor knows, the stomach symptom identified by the patient, is the homeostatic response to still some other problem. How could a mere mortal know for sure?

While it would be convenient to judge chiropractic on the basis of an "average" patient and construct research projects from this perspective, it would overlook the uniqueness of patients. Remember the admittance several years ago that the accepted 98.6 degrees Fahrenheit considered normal had been disproved? What accounts for the wide range of cholesterol levels having little to do with longevity or overall health? We are each so different, an attempt to create predictable models from within the bias of traditional research may be impossible.

Meanwhile, the name calling and infighting continues. Like the brave test pilots who noticed the extreme vibration of their aircraft before breaking through the sound barrier, chiropractic is simultaneously experiencing entropy from the diminished insurance money available and political infighting stemming from philosophical differences. As outside influences continue to pummel the profession, these internally destabilizing aspects of chiropractic are likely to harm the advancement of the profession more than ever.

Paradoxically, what is splitting the profession apart is an unwavering commitment by both factions to protect chiropractic! The Scientists want to safeguard the profession from what they perceive as religious zealots who use questionable or unproven approaches with patients. The Philosophers want to protect the profession from being relegated to a non-invasive therapy for the treatment of low back pain. While the most articulate and passionate of both factions choose sides and battle it out, an overwhelming majority of the profession can see the truth in both ends of the spectrum and are quietly going about their practices. As this "tastes great—less filling" argument continues to consume the attentions of these self-appointed warriors, the profession sees a growing number of its ranks abandoning practice.

There is a simple cause and a simple solution to this distracting political standoff. While some might find the medicine too bitter or the side effects too drastic, the only reason why chiropractors have the luxury to divide themselves in this way is because of the influence of third party reimbursement! Apparently, "insurance equality" has created a major inequality in chiropractic.

Without the influence of third party reimbursement, chiropractic would have probably long ago mended the straight/mixer argument, since "how" one helps a patient is seemingly less divisive than "why" one helps a patient. The science/philosophy argument more deeply divides the profession because it is a metaphor for our individual religious faith, belief structure, world view, and the ability to trust our five senses. From the bloody crusades of the medieval period to the more recent episode of "ethnic cleansing", millions have sacrificed their lives in the lofty pursuit of "protecting the world from the scourge of _____." You fill in the blank.

Remove all forms of third party reimbursement and this problem would disappear overnight. Require doctors, regardless of their scientific or philosophical bent, to present their case in the unencumbered free marketplace without the involvement of insurance companies, IMEs, HMOs, or government purse strings, and the whole practice landscape simplifies. Coexistence will be much more tolerable. Then, we can judge each other on the value we respectively add to the universe, instead of how much money one makes or how Dr. SoAndSo may be "polluting the profession."

Ironically, just as Aristotle was quoted as saying, "Look to the spine" to uncover the source of ill health, today, those who look to the spine merely need to "Follow the money" to uncover the source of ill health in chiropractic. ■

LURKING THROUGH LIFE

In the 1960s, at the height of the cold war, government officials devised a way to decentralize communications among vital organizations and government agencies. Fearing that strategic removal of traditional communication channels would cripple the United States during a national emergency, the Internet was created.

This giant web of interconnected computers spanned the globe using high speed electronic communications. Digital messages were broken up into bite-sized "packets" of information and sent at high speed between "nodes" of the network. If one or many nodes were damaged, off-line, or sabotaged, messages could still be routed through still other interconnected computer sites so the message would reach its target. Later, to share time on high speed supercomputers, colleges and universities joined this affiliation of computers. This allowed access to computer files, databases, and other information anywhere in the world from a computer and a phone line. With the expansion of commercial on-line computer services such as American On Line, CompuServe, and others, private citizens have access to this incredible array of computer services.

Besides access to data, on-line services have created forums for people around the world with similar interests to communicate with each other. You can think of these interest groups or "newsgroups" as a lot like a hotel lobby, full of people talking with each other. It's better than the lobby of a hotel because instead of just tuning into the conversation with the people in your immediate proximity, you can read the conversations of everyone in the room. But of course there isn't an actual room—everyone's sharing the same computer screen!

At any given time, there can be as many as 20 or more people in the same "room." Not everyone is talking (writing) at the same time. There are some people who never contribute anything to the conversations. Because this passive behavior is so common, these voyeurs have a name. In cyberspace parlance, these people are called lurkers.

Are you a lurker?

Many people I meet are lurking their way through life. They sit on the sidelines, quietly observing, waiting for conclusions and outcomes to be decided for them. These meek sheep are afraid to take a stand, express an opinion, or assume a leadership position. Imagine how this lack of confidence is perceived by patients! Just imagine how this impedes the healing process and causes a patient to question their decision to consult a chiropractor!

Lurkers lack the self-confidence to contribute or ask questions at seminars. Lurkers avoid confronting a staff member who is sabotaging the practice.

Lurkers want everyone to like them.

A lurking chiropractor is almost an oxymoron. After all, they've chosen a profession that mainstream society believes doesn't work, isn't necessary, and is basically a scam. If being liked was so important, other career choices would have been much more fulfilling. Psychologists suggest that the real dynamic at play here, the mother of all fears, is the fear of abandonment.

As a four- or five-year old, I remember walking out on a pier with my parents. This wooden structure jutted out into the Pacific ocean, somewhere in the Long Beach or Santa Monica, California area. I don't remember the specific circumstances but I remember that I wanted to stop, but my parents didn't, and they continued walking down the boardwalk. This was a traumatic, life-shaping experience. Perhaps you don't even remember your abandonment experience(s). But the possibility of being abandoned by our parents, and then later by friends at school, and then patients or staff members, has caused each of us to adopt various coping strategies. Some of us shrink into the background and become the wallflower. Others, over-compensate, assuming a loud, "life of the party" posture. Still others secretly attempt to undermine authority, breaking the rules and vandalizing the world around them. The low self-esteem that provides the catalyst for these and other abandonment coping strategies severely hinders the doctor/patient relationship. Combine them with a fascination with the diagnostic and technical aspects of chiropractic, and you have a doctor who is lurking in his or her own office!

If you recognize that lurking is costing you your practice and your life, and you want to turn things around, here are some suggestions from a former lurker:

1. Become internally directed. One of the processes of successful childhood is moving away from being externally directed, to being internally directed. The tumultuous time of adolescence is the testing ground for this disengagement from our parents (external), to self-reliance as a healthy adult. Too bad it coincides with massive hormonal changes and embarrassing skin conditions! So instead of emerging from this period and listening to our own voice, many simply go from the external control of parents, to the external control of a social group. While teens may talk about individuality, they dress alike. They may wish to make their unique mark, but they listen to the same music. So much for individuality!

Later as doctors, these same individuals get subluxations looking over their shoulders at the chiropractor down the street. What will the other chiropractors say? What would my patients think? Innovation is halted. New ideas are ignored. No one wants to be first.

Action step: Develop a mission statement or statement of purpose. Build your own internal benchmarks and guidance systems. Clearly articulate your reason for existence. Why were you put here? Who do you want to work with? What result or outcomes do you want to occur by contributing through chiropractic? What do you want your tombstone to read? Do your homework!

2. Recognize opinions are cheap. The universe puts the least value on things that are the most common and abundant. Sand is cheap. Pennies are cheap. Air is cheap. Opinions like the ones I'm expressing here are cheap also. Like everyone else with an opinion, I just made it up. I invented it. It's just my opinion.

Those who are the loudest, most vocal, most dogmatic, and least open to opposing ideas or viewpoints, are often the least secure in the point of view they've adopted. This lack of security is often displayed by doctors who become professional students, taking themselves away from the demands of their families, so as to acquire still more initials after their names. In the misguided notion that even still more education will solve the problems they face, these doctors become intimidated by what they don't know.

Action step: No one has a corner on the truth. I certainly don't. Perhaps you should stop taking your opinions and those of others so seriously. Let someone else be "right" next time. The value and effectiveness of your opinions are not dependent upon them being mirrored by anyone else. I'm reminded of a quip made by Johnny Carson about one his wives, "If you both agree on everything, one of you is unnecessary."

3. Expose yourself to more risks. One of the most unsettling feelings among lurkers is the ambiguity that results from risk-taking. Again, this is a self-confidence issue. Without experience in taking risks, there is uncertainty in being able to effectively predict the outcome of making a particular choice. Without the assurance of a "sure thing," one's energy is spent trying to sustain the status quo. Change becomes terrifying. Decision making is put off. Control and direction of one's future is in the hands of others.

Action step: Breaking this debilitating behavior starts with recognizing it, and then slowly taking more risks. Start with small, inconsequential risks. Try out new tastes, new clothes, and new ways of speaking. You can begin this process without anyone else even knowing what you're doing. As you "raise the bar" and take increasingly riskier stands and behaviors you'll notice that no one else really cares! What you really discover is that your little reality of what's "right" and what's "wrong" is entirely a mental construct! Not only can this realization be incredibly liberating, it can cause you to laugh at yourself for waiting so long to enjoy the fresh air outside your little cocoon!

It's ironic that as much as lurkers hope to be correct, liked, and accepted, the more they wimp out and evade taking a stand, the less likely they are to be correct, liked and accepted. It's tempting for leaders to consult the latest polling data and test their ideas with "trial balloons." However, that's not leadership, that's a popularity contest. The most effective leaders are not always liked, but they are almost always respected. If it comes to choosing one over the other, I'll take respect! ■

JUST SAY NO

The thought is so disgusting it's hard to see the logic behind it. The notion is so out of character with the fundamental basis of chiropractic it's difficult to understand. And the danger is so great it's urgent that every chiropractor step forward. Is it AIDS? No. Is it thousands of new students competing for your patients? No. Is it a new managed care scheme? No. It's the growing faction within chiropractic that wants to see an expansion of chiropractic into the dispensing of pharmaceuticals!

It's hard to believe, but in more and more states there has been a movement that is vocal and increasingly adamant, demanding the "right" to administer certain drugs and potions. These can be powerful and politically savvy chiropractors who see the direction towards drugs as the ultimate in one-stop patient service. Others apparently seek ways to blur the distinction between medicine and chiropractic in the hopes of gaining acceptance, validation, or income. Whatever the motive, it is vitally important that every chiropractor reject these moves and maintain the purity of chiropractic. I'd like to propose four reasons why:

Chiropractors aren't trained to administer drugs. As a practical matter, current chiropractic training doesn't cover the prescription of drugs. If it were legal, you can be sure weekend seminar courses would spring up to answer the demand. Learning the use and contraindications of the typical handful of commonly prescribed drugs would probably be relatively easy. But, that would be like thinking that knowing how to move bones is all it takes to become a chiropractor!

Perhaps one of the motives for the inclusion of drugs in the chiropractic repertoire is to remove a perceived barrier to chiropractors being "gatekeepers" in a managed care arena. Either you are a masochist who enjoys the already intrusive amounts of paperwork and accountability to third parties, or you simply despise your low malpractice insurance premiums. Which is it?

Prescribing drugs smells of the Faustian deal osteopaths must have made with medicine.

Chiropractic doesn't need any more enemies. As this movement gains momentum from chiropractors who haven't a clue as to the potential long range damage, it will awaken a sleeping dog that lost much of its bite when the Wilk's case settled in federal court. If you think the medical community will sit back and allow chiropractic intrusion into their domain, you're either self-administering some controlled substances, crazy, or both.

Remember those chiropractic forefathers who went to jail for "practicing medicine without a license?" In all too many states, the very laws that enable chiropractic to co-exist with medicine, specifically include assurances of the fundamental difference between medicine and chiropractic, and a respect for those boundaries. Attempting to modify this arrangement, even in the most subtle way, will unleash an attack that will make the *Wall Street Journal* article, the ABC *20/20* television story, and the *Consumer Reports* profile look like endorsements for chiropractic!

What if the shoe was on the other foot? What if the medical profession decided it wanted to add spinal adjustments to its little black bag of tricks. How would you feel about that?

Even with the apparent "successes" of certain medicines and the consumer convenience offering pharmaceuticals would bring, chiropractic would invite the wrath of a well-funded adversary that is simply waiting for an excuse to don the boxing gloves again.

Chiropractic philosophy rejects the use of drugs. Some might think this is the weakest argument, but I think it's one of the strongest.

Those who reject the Ten Commandments simply because they are old, or have fallen under the spell of scientism, may find this perspective the most difficult to understand.

Chiropractic was founded on several fundamental truths, that in our haste to become accepted, validated, or simply make car payments, are easily overlooked. You know, like the power that made the body heals the body. Like, doctors don't heal, only the body (without interference) can heal itself. Like, chiropractors treat the person, not the disease. Like, chiropractors treat the cause, not the symptoms. While it may seem expedient, the use of drugs goes against everything chiropractic has stood for since 1895.

If you truly want to administer drugs and you see it as the key to patient satisfaction and the salvation of your practice, there's a wonderful way you can do it without bastardizing chiropractic or tampering with the scope of practice laws. It is so elegant and so obvious that it's easy to overlook: become a medical doctor!

If becoming a medical doctor requires too much work, then maybe you're not as committed to this precept as you thought. Perhaps like your patients, you want results the easy way, without personal responsibility or effort.

If you want to prescribe drugs, this also might be a good year to dance on Harvey Lilliard's and D. D. Palmer's graves.

Chiropractic must remain separate and distinct. State legislatures and even the federal government have already admonished the profession when it presents diverse and conflicting points of view. Some states have as many as three and four different chiropractic associations, societies, and splinter groups, plus an alarming number of apathetic doctors who don't participate at all. When these different lobbyists show up at the capitol, the wisest legislators throw up their hands and require the profession to get its act together and present a unified message. Good advice.

Worse, when you combine medicine with chiropractic you confuse patients. Like the chiropractor who administers physical therapy in the absence of sufficient patient education, patients are unsure whether the "shock therapy" or the doctor's adjustments are the cause of their health restoration. Blurring this difference, simply hoping the patient will make the chiropractor the hero in the whole pain relief experience, is an egotistical and obscene motive that reveals true insecurity.

Maybe the real root of this movement is the notion that results alone are king. Perhaps it is simply playing out the age old question of the ends justifying the means. Or, is the administering of a drug to speed up, slow down, or numb the body simply a misguided attempt to please and be liked by the patient?

As the practice of chiropractic becomes increasingly challenging, you'll see continued efforts to drift towards the belief that prescribing drugs will save chiropractic. And while it might save an individual practice, it will destroy chiropractic. Treating symptoms such as the lack of new patients or the lack of validation and acceptance is a bankrupt idea. Trumpeting the addition of drugs as a way to serve patients better is a dangerous game of self-deception. ■

ARE WE
DRUGLESS OR NOT?

To merge or not to merge? Mercy or no mercy? Compromise or adapt? As the intraprofessional squabbles continue, more and more chiropractors concerned about the increasing bashing of chiropractic by managed care organizations and the media, are wondering why chiropractic can't unite under a single banner. It will require just such a collaboration and united front to sharpen the impact and influence of chiropractic. As chiropractors put fellow chiropractors in their respective gun sights, singling them out as the devil incarnate and responsible for their lack of new patients, reduced income, and battles with cost-cutting bureaucrats, chiropractic continues to be assailed.

Besides the necessary leadership to turn the tide and unite the many ardent and vocal factions within chiropractic, it will require the rank and file of the chiropractic profession to agree upon what they do. Based upon the observation that it is the rare patient who knows what his or her chiropractor does, it's likely that few chiropractors can clearly articulate the unique domain and focus of their practice!

All too many chiropractors, when asked by a new acquaintance what they do, they simply reply, "I'm a chiropractor." After all, it's easy, it's so simple, and doesn't require much thought. Most everyone has heard about chiropractors, so, few push further, asking for a more in depth explanation. Whew! How lucky can you get? That way you don't have to wrangle with the importance of the nervous system, its protective covering, the effect of spinal malfunction, and the technical aspects of your adjusting approach. "I'm a chiropractor." While this is convenient, your new friend simply applies everything they've ever heard about chiropractors, to you. Unfortunately, their baggage and perceptions may not be especially flattering!

When this lazy, vague, shorthand way of describing what you do is extrapolated by the dozens or more chiropractors in a given town or city, you have an entire community that is unsure what chiropractic is or what chiropractors do. When you multiply these unfocused doctors in a city, by the sometimes hundreds of cities in a state, you have an entire state divided against itself. The result? Some states with as many as three or four associations, societies, or ad hoc groups of doctors. No wonder state legislators are confused and managed care organizations are quick to take advantage! Then, combine these many fragmented states and you have an entire country of chiropractors who practically invite abuse and disparaging press.

Clearly, I am not the first person to observe the futility of the current situation. This battle has raged since the very beginning when even father and son could not agree on a vision for chiropractic. Perhaps it is unwise, but I'd like to take an inventory of what we *can* agree upon and ascertain the choke point; the compressive lesion; the subluxation, if you will, of a lack of "ease" within the profession.

Can we agree that chiropractic deals with bones and nerves? Hope so. Can we agree that chiropractic doctors locate areas of spinal malfunction and its many possible associated affects or manifestations on the body? Can we agree that chiropractic doctors attempt to reduce these malfunctions by restoring motion or improved structure to these aberrant spinal areas? So far so good?

Now, for what I'm told may be more difficult. Can we agree that only the body has the capacity to heal itself and that no doctor of any kind, type, technique, or political persuasion has ever healed a patient, and that only a patient, with the unleashing of its inborn potential to be healthy, can heal?

Further, that because proper health requires proper function, and that only the body can heal itself and doesn't need any help-just no interference, can we all agree that chiropractic is a drugless healing art?

I'm told that the barrier to professional unity is the use of the word "drugless." Here's why it is essential that we agree on using this word (or its equivalent) if we want to unite the profession and assume our rightful place:

1. Legal distinction. This may be difficult for doctors who were not thrown into jail "for practicing medicine without a license" or who are relatively new doctors and assume their right to practice chiropractic is guaranteed by their creator. The licensing of chiropractors in many states and jurisdictions was based upon the unique healing approach used by chiropractic that did not compete with medicine. It was this distinction that permitted chiropractic to exist in the first place! Blurring the line between chiropractic and medicine, simply for the right to recommend an over-the-counter analgesic or receive hospital privileges, intrudes upon the already tenuous "demilitarized zone" separating allopathic medicine from chiropractic. How would you feel if the tables were turned and medical doctors suddenly recognized what chiropractors have known for a century? I can see it now, "Receive chiropractic-like adjustments in the safety and convenience of your family physician's office. Covered by your HMO! Approved by Medicare! Special introductory offer! Call for an appointment today!"

2. Confuses the patient. Worse than blurring the distinctions between medicine and chiropractic, it makes it more difficult to demonstrate the competitive advantage of being a "drug-free alternative" to medical care. Like children who face the ambiguity of "good" drugs (from the doctor) and "bad" drugs (from the dealer on the playground), adults, who in growing numbers are abandoning traditional medical protocols, will become increasingly confused. More and more of the baby boom generation aren't falling for the knee-jerk prescriptions. They're seeing their aging parents pumped up on drugs, who take still other drugs to overcome the side effects of the first drugs, who receive still more drugs to deal with the new side effects...

3. Propagates a lie. While the jury continues to debate the alleged efficacy of artificial immunizations and we continue to encounter an increasing number of antibiotic-resistant viruses, the world is watching. Symptom treating is counterproductive whether it's treating the symptom of a disease state in the body, or the symptoms of poor business planning or child rearing. When chiropractors stick to their guns by being focused on "cause," they are abiding by a universal truth that will ultimately be rewarded. Some may be impatient for the rewards sure to accrue to one who is faithful to the truth, but our generation may not be the one to reap and enjoy this accepted leadership role. (Based upon the lies and convenient oversights of what our children are learning in grade school, the next generation is likely to be deeply entrenched in symptom treating, too.) Remember, the truth can set you free!

4. Avoids confrontation. Ironically, getting the right to discuss drug use with chiropractic patients or simply shunning the "drugless" label as being too restrictive, is the result of succumbing to the temptress of leadership: wanting to be liked. It's not like the most conservative chiropractors claim, that proponents of drugs and therapy are just frustrated medical doctors. While that's a convenient argument, the truth is more likely that a large number of them simply want to fit in. It's not particularly fun to be the eternal "nerd" of the health care profession. But leadership is not the result of putting your wet finger in the air, or taking an opinion poll to find out what is most expedient. Leadership means taking some arrows and standing up for what is right, even if it is unpopular. Apparently some in chiropractic aren't truly prepared for a leadership role. Perhaps being a victim and garnering strength by being against the establishment is as much of a stand as we can expect from a generation of chiropractors weaned on easy insurance money.

Whichever political group wins, those in a leadership position in the losing camp, with its power and influence, will lose their jobs. Certainly we all want to be liked and it's not a crime to desire acceptance, but attempting to expand the scope of practice or sell out chiropractic to short term "me-tooism" has fatal consequences. Unfortunately, while the doctors squabble over turf or who is more right, the patient is now in critical condition! ■

CREATING YOUR
DREAM PRACTICE

At a time when countless chiropractors are focused on surviving, it may seem like the wrong time to dream a big dream and redesign your practice. However, today's changing practice climate represents an exciting opportunity to rethink your practice and align it with your purpose and vision.

Today is the perfect time to make a change. Your next new patient to show up is the perfect time to make a change. The next patient you touch would be an excellent time to make a change. If you wait until you know enough, have enough money, have enough time, or the arrangement of the planets is somehow perfect, you've succumbed to the fear of the unknown that naturally accompanies any kind of change.

Time is the only resource that each, regardless of our knowledge, financial accomplishments, or practice size, is given in perfectly equal measure. What separates a practice that is thriving, from a practice that is floundering is rarely talent, location, experience, procedures, technique, or whether they adjust on the first visit. The most obvious difference is how each respective practitioner uses his or her time. Not necessarily the amount of time spent with each patient, but how their time is spent when they aren't even seeing patients!

How do you spend your time?

Do you squander your valuable time resources eavesdropping on inane plots and the mutually exchanged insults of situational TV comedies? Do you vicariously pretend to be a star running back, wasting your precious moments watching ESPN? If your practice isn't what you think it should be or could be, these and other thoughtless uses of your time are luxuries you can't afford. Remember that your practice is a direct reflection of what and how you think. If you're not thinking; if you're numbing yourself with television or some other distraction, take the first step necessary to relaunch your practice by taking a vacation... from your TV set!

The fact is, most practices are the same as other practices, give or take 20%. This is probably because most doctors read the same chiropractic magazines, go to the same chiropractic seminars, and learn the same basic adjusting techniques. When you recognize the stunning similarities among most practices, the notion of chiropractors being controversial, off-the-wall renegades becomes almost laughable! Fitting in seems more important. Being liked seems somehow necessary. Going along to get along has become the rule. What ever happened to the chiropractic warriors? Where have all the chiropractors gone who wanted to make waves and generally irritate the medical community? Did easy insurance money tame them? Have hospital privileges tempted them? Has a big mortgage payment scared them off?

If you're still trying to apply procedures, paperwork, and patient protocols from the previous decade (or before), you already have a grasp of the disorienting change that is occurring. As with any endeavor, your brain will be your most potent instrument in your mastery of change. But like the famous computer adage, "garbage in, garbage out," your brain can't help you if it's not stimulated with fresh input. Consider one or more of the following:

1. Admit there's a problem. Many doctors are still in denial, unwilling to even acknowledge times have changed. You can watch them in seminars, still looking for the spoon-fed, step-by-step procedures; a recipe book of someone else's thinking! How many seminars does it take to realize that practice is a performance. You can't have the practice described from the seminar platform unless, and until, you *think* like the seminar speaker. There are no shortcuts. If you share different values, if your personality significantly differs, if your belief and understanding of chiropractic is divergent, or if your passion and energy level is anemic, you will never get the same results. Ever.

2. Understand the problem. Understandably, when many people face a challenge, they are tempted to run from it or ignore it. However, it's been my experience that the solutions to most problems are likely to be found in the vicinity of the problems. The solution to a new patient problem is most likely to be found amongst the new patients who *do* make it in. Solving a compliance problem can often be traced to a better understanding of why some patients *do* comply. Questions about financial policy are best answered where and when patients pay for their care. Instead of running from the issue, or numbing yourself with TV, food, exercise, sex, or some other distraction, get as close to the problem as you can. That's most likely where the answers are.

3. Remember your philosophy. One of the most valuable things I have obtained from my work in chiropractic has been the acquisition of a personal philosophy that is constantly seeking "cause." No longer am I tempted by symptom-treating solutions to yard maintenance, car repair, interpersonal relationships, or any other interaction, disappointment, or situation. A willingness to continually question the status quo can be a particularly helpful skill if you want to facilitate change. Start by questioning why you take your current route to the office and then proceed through every function, every procedure, every scrap of paper you touch, to everything you say and do. Why are you doing it that way? There may be perfectly good explanations, but make it a habit to regularly hold everything to the test of relevancy and accountability.

4. Talk to other practitioners. Break the cycle of your chiropractic funnel vision by getting out of your normal circle of friends. Know any other licensed professionals? Dentists? Architects? Veterinarians? Accountants? Cross-fertilize your brain by sharing ideas, procedures, and the unique challenges of other types of practices. How do they handle collections, new patients, staff hiring, vacations, marketing communications, paperwork, and other issues. You'll be astonished how many things you can learn from professionals in other disciplines that haven't been mutated by your chiropractic subculture or years of in-line breeding at chiropractic seminars!

5. Read some non-chiropractic books. Reading nonfiction is the best way to create new neural pathways in the brain. Learn about customer service strategies from Japan, the fast-food industry, or the automotive field. Read what the mainstream business community is doing to adapt to the same sort of changes you're facing. Books by Naisbit, Toffler, Peters, Popcorn, Townsend, and others can spark countless adaptations for your practice. Don't wait for a television documentary! The good ideas are in books. Not a reader? Many of the best books have been placed on audio cassette. You're not still listening to the radio on your drive to work are you?

6. Write it down. One of the most powerful ways to solve problems, imprint solutions, and create a new vision for your practice is to begin an aggressive journaling program. You're reading my journal now. This is how I organize my thoughts, determine what I believe about a particular topic, and generally rehearse my brain. Instead of 1300 word essays, maybe what you're looking for is an opportunity to think on paper and focus the vision you have for your practice. Sadly, all too many doctors can better describe what they *don't* want their practices to be, than precisely what they *do* want them to be! If the future of your practice is merely a vague longing, an incomplete yearning, or a dream that is blurry and out of focus, you'll never achieve the greatness you deserve. If you will muster the discipline and use your journal to describe in excruciating detail what you want, it can be yours.

7. Take small risks. Attempt to eat an entire submarine sandwich in a single bite, and you're likely to choke. Same with integrating change in your practice. Too much change too quickly can put it into shock. Yet taking big risks is rarely the problem. The problem is quitting too soon. Like the child gardener who keeps pulling up the seeds to see if they've sprouted, many doctors stop implementing a procedure or policy or piece of paperwork just before it can pay off! Doctors who seek instant gratification, or who have an unrealistic notion of how long it takes to see results, are often the ones who become seminar "junkies." While their thirst for the latest information is legendary, they often fail to implement anything successfully because they either lack the necessary discipline or are too impatient. Even patients can tell, remarking, "Looks like the doctor's been to another one of those seminars..."

It's time to make change. The world will never be the same and the soil is ripe for planting. Planting the wrong seeds at the wrong time of the year is foolish and invites disappointment. Those who recognize the beginnings of spring have pulled the weeds from the soil of opportunity and are sowing for the harvest. Wishful thinking will not change the season. And waiting even longer simply risks missing another harvest. ■

BE CAREFUL!

"Be careful," your mom warned as you left for school each morning. "Be careful," you were warned as you left on your first date. "Be careful," your chemistry teacher warned you at the beginning of a new experiment. "Be careful," you were warned when adjusting patients. Be careful. Repeated by generation after generation, it's a mantra that ranks up there with "Have a nice day." Maybe that's the problem with your practice—you're just too darned careful!

Reminding ourselves and our children to be careful suggests that there is reason to fear the world. It suggests a malevolent, rather than a benevolent world view. It suggests the world "out there" is dangerous and, that if we're not careful, we'll become hapless victims of the world, both human and natural.

Careful people don't get much done. They worry a lot. They fret. They play games of "what if" in which they imagine themselves the victims of everything from the shame of bankruptcy, to the scorn of the Joneses down the street. If these intellectual dress rehearsals don't become self-fulfilling prophecies, they at least hold countless people in the bondage of fear.

Run down a mental list of the most influential inventors, leaders, and scholars the world has ever known, and you won't find too many "careful" personalities on your list. There have been millions of careful bureaucrats. But the people who make things happen and make a mark, either in their families, communities, or the human history of the world, aren't the careful type. They may have left the house without their coats, stayed up too late, missed some meals, and generally embraced life with reckless abandonment. Their personal conviction and determination propelled them into the spotlight. They boldly took a stand, and swayed others in the process. Being careful limits one's performance to the tested, the average, and the mediocre.

When we get goose bumps from the performance of a great musician, or when our eyes mist with tears from a touching moment, or when we experience an adrenaline rush of purpose and motivation, being careful is the furthest thing from our minds. We are inspired by those willing to surrender to the moment; to risk hitting the high note; to stand in the path of an on-coming tank. When we see others take great risks, especially those that fly in the face of conventional wisdom or political correctness, we too, are inspired to soar to new heights.

Been doing any soaring recently?

One of the fears that can consume some practitioners is that of malpractice. After the years of study, personal sacrifice, and making a great living, many doctors are so fearful of losing what they have, that they become spineless cowards. So afraid of what the doctor down the street will think, they put off the implementation of cutting edge ideas. Fearful of making a mistake, countless doctors are paralyzed into inaction. Worse, terrified of what they may find, they avoid the self-study and introspection required to find the causal roots of their own fears. Their "carefulness" has created a straitjacket whose straps are only loosened when the pain of inaction eclipses the fear of the unknown.

It is tempting when embarking on a new project, meeting a new patient, or trying a new procedure, to hedge our bets. Holding back, just a little, so in case it doesn't work we can save face. "I didn't think it would work, anyway," we say to ourselves, validating our fears and justifying our failure.

It's when we hold back that we almost assure failure.

Many historians believe Israel's success in the 1967 war was due largely because they had so much to lose. Their enemies were fighting for an idea—but Israel was fighting for its life! The fiercest battles (and the increased likelihood of success) are conducted by those who have no other means of escape. Total commitment is required. Somehow, we don't seem to fight as vigorously when there is a back door through which we can escape. Holding back; being too careful, creates a doorway that sabotages our resolve, sealing our fates in the status quo.

Plus, being careful makes us too self-conscious. Not only is it unnatural to become aware of every word we speak and every movement of our bodies, it practically invites failure. It is during this self-consciousness that we are most likely to "choke." You've seen this occur when a valued ballplayer suddenly finds himself in a batting slump, or when a "successful" doctor discovers his or her new patient statistics are in a nose dive. It is only when ballplayers or doctors detach themselves (their egos) from their performances, that they can get out of the way of themselves. It's no time to be careful!

1. Get some new stimulation. It's impossible to drink from an empty well, so nurture your most important asset in all of this; your brain. Time to spend a day in a museum. Time to visit the magazine rack at the bookstore. Time to take a tour of a local factory. You get the picture—stimulate your cerebral cortex by focusing on something that doesn't have any direct correlation with your practice or the problem at hand. Ask questions. Become so immersed in your experience that you forget about yourself. While those who are always seeking control will shrink from the seemingly lack of practical value of this exercise, it's exactly what's needed. You'll be surprised how your optimism will improve and how you'll be able to see your challenges from a fresh perspective. Stop thinking about yourself!

2. Take risks in other areas of your life. Increase your confidence and raise your risk tolerance by embracing non-practice related areas of growth. For some this may be as easy as wearing a necktie that is just a little bolder than you're normally comfortable with. Or purchasing a car that isn't quite as practical as your conscious tells you it should be. Or taking a different way to work. Or going out for Thai, Indian, or some other type of exotic food that you've never had before. (Remember, whole cultures have survived for years eating this stuff!) Your mission is to become less careful and invite whatever happens to happen. It's called life! Get out of the safe, predictable, and claustrophobic box you've created for yourself.

3. Abandon your goals. There is nothing scarier than reaching your goals. It produces a lethargy that is hard to shake. Succeeding in the goals of being accepted at chiropractic college, graduating, passing the boards, opening your practice, getting patients, surviving, growing, and thriving have put many doctors on a path to... well, boredom. Instead of being focused on the next rung of the success ladder (getting a diplomate, being accepted into the local HMO, hospital privileges, owning a Lexus, etc.), take a deep breath and enjoy life. Take some time off. Get a hobby. Get reacquainted with your family. Your practice will still be there! Remember, we are most likely to lose that which we hold onto the tightest.

Of course at the root of this notion of being careful, is the sad attempt at avoiding making a mistake. Sad, because it is only in risking the "making of a mistake" that progress and growth is achieved. Just imagine if D. D. Palmer had been too careful with Harvey Lilliard. Being careful, being right, or even being popular, holds little hope of producing the breakthroughs, accomplishment, and fulfillment for which we each secretly yearn. ■

THREE CLUES

I used to collect baseball cards. Yes, I was one of those tragic cases whose mom discarded thousands of cards, which today would bring six figures at any card swap. What's sad isn't the financial loss, but the loss of the important institution those baseball cards documented: the classic New York Yankees.

Yes, the Yankees are still here, but the powerhouse line-up of a Mickey Mantle, Yogi Berra, Roger Maris, Whitey Ford, and Joe Peppitone are gone for good. Free agents changed all that. Free agency helped level the playing field and distributed baseball talent among various teams much differently than in the good old days. Now, professional baseball teams are generally so equally mediocre, I've lost any desire to keep up with the players. Just as baseball has changed, so too has the chiropractic practice.

To get a glimpse of the future of chiropractic, have a look back to the pre-insurance equality days of the 1960s for clues. What did it take to make it back then?

Clue #1

Outgoing personality. It wasn't too long ago that you could learn a couple of adjusting techniques, do some advertising, hire someone to process insurance with a computer, and you could be a "success." Countless "technique nerds" with their spartan, low-overhead offices and bookish tableside manners were able to help lots of patients enjoy a taste of neuromuscular-skeletal chiropractic. As a monument to this exciting time, their trophy cases of inactive patient files were bulging and their reception rooms were empty. Clearly the relationship was just physical, never reaching the intellectual, much less the emotional or spiritual dimensions necessary for long-term patient retention.

If you're introverted or analytical or uncomfortable with the ambiguities of interacting with patients, the future of your career is dependent upon making some personality changes! Like evaluating a patient's health complaint, it's helpful to approach the cause, and avoid symptom treating.

Self-esteem. This is the mother of all personality dysfunctions. Raise your self-worth by reviewing the case files of hopeless patients who began care in your office, but regained their lives through your efforts. What's been your success rate? Is it 80%? How about 90%? Higher? You're good! Start believing it.

Appearance. Feeling kinda geeky? Wearing pocket protectors? A polyester lab coat? Five-year old shoes? Maybe it's time for a makeover. It's too bad that results don't speak for themselves, but we've become a culture sensitive to brand names, designer labels, and appearances. It may not seem practical, or you may feel uncomfortable spending money on your wardrobe, but face it, patients want to associate with a successful looking doctor.

Technical certainty. How many more journals must you read before you feel comfortable with your ability to help patients? How many more adjusting techniques must you dabble with to feel proficient? If you're into structure, take those post X-rays. If you're into function, perform the needed orthopedic tests at regular progress examinations. Get the "technical" out of the way so you can concentrate on personal skills necessary to truly connect with your patients.

Acceptance. If you're so worried about people liking you, why did you choose chiropractic? Or did you forget? You're supposed to be pushing the envelope and making people feel uncomfortable. Your job is to help patients question the status quo and disrupt their wrong-headed thinking. I bet the teachers back in college who, in retrospect, were the most influential, made you mad, uncomfortable, guilty, and pushed you to your limits. Now, it's your job to do that to your patients!

Results are not enough. Doctors who are thriving in today's

deregulated chiropractic environment have personalities that attend to the emotional and spiritual needs of their patients, with the same ease with which they address the physical needs of their patients.

Clue #2

Family practice. Dissect the successful practice of the 1960s and you'll find huge family practices. Families came in together, crowding into the adjusting room, arguing about who was going to get adjusted first. Going to the chiropractor was a family activity. You wouldn't think of leaving a family member at home!

Today, retooling your practice from a personal injury and worker's comp mill, into a place entire families would feel comfortable, may necessitate some changes.

Comfortable with children. It goes without saying that if you're not comfortable checking and adjusting children, entire families won't be showing up. This is a technical question as much as a personality question. Are children comfortable around you? Is your office full of scary Halloween bones and skeletons?

Family fees. The same holds true with fees. If you think patients will find it reasonable to pay $40 for an adjustment for each family member, you either need to move to Beverly Hills or start paying for the care you get for free! Family plans and other creative fee schedules are only possible after a total disengagement from the insurance industry and passing up the lucrative personal injury market. Sorry, but you're going to have to choose sides.

Patient education. Less obvious is the need for the very best patient education. In the 1960s, this almost always involved some form of spinal care class, lectures, or public speaking outreaches. Back then, before prompter-reading pretty boy television news anchors set such a high standard, lectures could be quite powerful. Today, back up your lectures with video, brochures, posters, "topics of the day," metaphors, power words, analogies, and other devices which use lots of pictures.

Clue #3

Cash practice. This is the most challenging aspect for doctors weaned on insurance. For many, the notion that patients would be inclined to pay for care out of their own pockets is inconceivable. However, not only were there incredibly successful cash-based practices in the 1960s, there are incredibly successful cash-based practices in the 1990s. In Australia, spinal manipulation rendered by medical doctors is covered under their national health insurance plan. Yet, chiropractic is thriving! True these doctors must deliver the goods, have personalities, and educate patients on the value of chiropractic, but most of the 2,000 chiropractors are enjoying a good living, sans the paperwork, second-guessing, and influence of third parties. It *can* be done. But who has the courage, discipline, and patient leadership skills to make it happen? Put all these issues together and a picture of the future starts to emerge. Those who are the deepest in denial will suggest this spartan view of the future flies in the face of the latest research affirming the success of chiropractic. Still others propose a different approach, trying to be more like medical doctors and hoping that acceptance can come without the price of being controlled by third parties. Live by the sword, die by the sword. How many times have you ever had your cake and eaten it too?

Each doctor will be asked to decide between the purity (and risk) of the doctor/patient relationship and the security (and control) of coming under the medical umbrella. Some will try to wait until the last minute before making their choice. Some will look over their shoulders to see how others decide. Still others will choose the path of least resistance, dooming the profession to the fate of osteopathy. What will it be? ■

PREACHING TO THE CHOIR

A profession of Lone Rangers like chiropractic will hopelessly remain splintered, and it's social impact blunted until chiropractors find themselves sharing similar experiences. Just as we accuse surgeons of seeing every problem requiring a surgical solution, the same tunnel vision is found in chiropractic. Upper cervical practitioners see every patient's problem as an upper cervical problem, just as every kinesiologist sees every patient's problem as a kinesiology problem. Liberals see the world requiring liberal solutions, and conservatives see the world as needing conservative solutions. Few can appreciate and embrace the truths found in the opposite extreme. The result is a profession with distracting infighting, dogmatic leadership, and a huge middle ground occupied by doctors uncertain, afraid, or unwilling to boldly proclaim the sometimes unpopular truth of chiropractic.

It's natural to associate with those who share a similar outlook on life, politics, child rearing, or some other issue. Rarely do we seek out those who hold perspectives opposite our own, or who ascribe to principles that threaten us. After recognizing our inability to change those who hold diametrically opposing viewpoints, we tend to settle into the safety of our respective subcultures to lick our wounds and seek renewal and affirmation from our like-minded peers. Instead of being broadened by divergent points of view, we are like the seven blind men, each touching different parts of an elephant, attempting to describe the entire elephant! Of course, a mitigating factor in all this is low self-esteem. When something that we make such an emotional investment in (such as our career, protocol, philosophy, technique, etc.) is attacked, *we* are attacked. That's why we defend our families, our homes, and our country. Confusing an adjusting technique with what chiropractic is all about, or thinking posture is more important than function (or vice versa!), or getting derailed by some narrow, dogmatic position that is an over-simplification. Worse, it produces a cranky, fixated chiropractor unable to adapt to today's rapidly changing practice environment.

When committing oneself to the Lone Ranger role of defending "truth, justice, and the American way," it makes it easier when there is an easily identified enemy. When the medical profession was the enemy, virtually every chiropractor could describe what they were against. Being against the same thing was unifying. But after the Wilk trial, the enemy became more obscure. The resulting "guerrilla war-fare" and hit and run tactics used by the medical underground (and its media accomplices) have muddied the waters. Canceling the office subscription to *Consumer's Report* or swearing off from watching ABC television after their airing of the *20/20* story (twice!) doesn't produce the same level of satisfaction as impugning the mechanistic mindset of a medic down the street! The solution? Attack your colleague across town who uses the XYZ technique, insult chiropractors who take 20 minutes with each patient, or who talk to their feet.

The point of course, is that chiropractic has little chance of assuming its rightful place until the petty turf wars of technique, philosophy, practice style, procedure, and other details are replaced by an agreement on the highest purposes of chiropractic.

This may be a lofty goal that will remain unattainable until a more deserving enemy can be broadly identified by the average chiropractor (managed care? the government? physical therapists?). Until then, what can be done?

1. Relicensure continuing education. The first step towards breaking down the barriers dividing the profession is to put doctors with differing viewpoints into the same room. State licensing boards can be instrumental in this effort, requiring attendance at annual programs in which intraprofessional issues are addressed, taught, and discussed. The leadership in each state must force the fringe, the wayward, and the weird out from underneath their respective rocks and into the sunlight. It's astonishing to me that there are still some states that do not require some type of mandatory, on-going continuing education program. Unless the profession steps forward to police itself, there will be others who will step in to fill the void.

2. Relevant continuing education. Those states which insist upon continuing education for relicensure are to be applauded. However, the quality of these programs leaves much to be desired. Many of these programs do little to uplift the profession or advance the crucial doctor/patient relationship. Instead, many doctors must endure esoteric presentations on mostly irrelevant topics that rarely supply usable information, encouragement, or practical action steps to improve patient care. Waiting until the last minute, doctors pack a two-day supply of newspapers, magazines, and unfinished paperwork to entertain themselves during the grueling weekend! The resulting "out-of-body-experience" is hardly life changing.

3. Attendance taking. Partly as a symptom of irrelevant programs, the best part of most association/society meetings takes place out in the hallways. Here, the good old boys can reminisce about the good old days and smoke cigarettes without judgmental stares. Worse than the missed opportunity to affirm and build up the membership, attendance must be monitored to assure everyone receives the required number of force-fed hours. While attendance is taken, fraud is rampant as associates sign in for each other or leave early! Why does this remind me of high school?

4. Standardize chiropractic college curricula. The next generation of chiropractors who will take the profession into its second century are in school now. Besides ringing up huge loans which could prompt individual decisions counterproductive to the future of the profession, these students are learning the bias and bigotry that continue to ostracize certain philosophical, diagnostic, and adjusting routines. While uniformity should not be the goal, colleges have the opportunity to nip these crippling attitudes in the bud. Unfortunately, all too many teachers are simply promulgating the same attitudes they were taught. Ending this inner-breeding could reduce intraprofessional jealousy and pointless counterproductive bickering.

5. Focus on the why, instead of the how. Maybe one way to help unify the profession would be a renewed emphasis on the "why" of chiropractic instead of the "how" of chiropractic. Sure, this would require a new level of maturity, but what publication, what organization, what school, what movement within chiropractic is willing to provide the necessary leadership to avoid the entropy that will lead to the self-destruction of this profession? Or, will market forces continue to assail the doctors walking around with the equivalent of "kick me" signs on their backs?

The number of chiropractors I meet who are dabbling in chiropractic, nutrition, naturopathy, homeopathy, and a variety of multi-level interests is a growing concern. Fashioning themselves as a modern D.D. Palmer, attempting to address the many facets of real health is a myth. Under the guise of "pulling from a variety of different disciplines to serve patients better," many of these doctors have become a jack-of-all-trades and a master of none. True, many health problems have physical, emotional, and spiritual components, but in this day and age, we are suspicious of the one-size-fits-all professional. How would you perceive an insurance salesman who also passes himself off as a financial planner, stock broker, futures trader, and real estate appraiser? How good at any one of these important professional roles could he or she be?

It is at the grass roots level that chiropractic must begin its housekeeping duties. Expecting national organizations to resolve these issues is merely wishful thinking. The future of chiropractic resides in the leadership and commitment exhibited at the local level. Just as we pretty much get the type of government we deserve, most doctors enjoy an influence in the healing arts at pretty much the level they deserve. If the status quo is acceptable, then no change is necessary. But if, on the other hand, after 100 years you'd thought chiropractic could be further along, then get involved. Your district and state association desperately need your help. ■

HALF EMPTY
OR HALF FULL?

Since 1981, when I first became a chiropractic patient, there have been some dramatic changes to the practice of chiropractic that will have an impact for many years to come. Unfortunately, many of these changes pose serious challenges. First, a review of what I think are the most significant developments of the last 10 or 15 years, and then why I'm optimistic about the future.

Erosion of indemnity insurance reimbursement. When I began chiropractic care, most people who were employed had some form of health insurance. These policies typically featured $100 deductibles and 80/20 coverage, serving to reduce the financial barrier to patients exploring the benefits of chiropractic care. Until it was outlawed, many chiropractors reduced this barrier further by offering care with no out-of-pocket expenses. This, combined with free spinal exams, huge yellow page ads, and a proliferation of management firms that taught doctors how to fully exploit a patient's insurance coverage, created a drunken stupor that many chiropractors are just now sobering up from.

Doctors who practiced during this period have been led to believe that free-flowing insurance money was normal. Yet, within the 100 year history of chiropractic, insurance is but a temporary diversion; a wonderful windfall. As much as some want to deny it, 1986 isn't coming back. Ever.

Growing pull towards headaches and low back pain. Led by the growing influence of scientism (if you can't taste it, touch it, measure it—it doesn't exist), many within chiropractic are reducing

223

their practices to the treatment of low back pain and headaches. Overlooking the scope of practice laws that permit chiropractic to even exist, many practitioners are ignoring the whole body phenomenon of the subluxation in favor of the easiest, most obvious neuromuscular-skeletal problems. Yes, chiropractic can be quite helpful with headaches and low back pain, however, putting chiropractic into such a small box tends to minimize the profound role of the nervous system.

Those who need research to prove chiropractic's vitalistic legacy are unlikely to find enough of it. If a century of anecdotal results isn't good enough for you, and you haven't experienced the far-reaching effects yourself, then search for double blind clinical trials that prove chiropractic works. While you're at it, why not search for proof that no two snowflakes are alike! Meanwhile, your colleagues recognize that "the doctor walks in with the patient" and are busy helping improve spinal structure and function, restoring a patient's inborn healing ability.

Rising debt loads among new graduates. As the standards of a chiropractic education continue to rise, so too has the cost. More and more new graduates are emerging from chiropractic college with a debt load approaching six figures! Defaults are likely to increase as chiropractic case averages rarely approach a patient's $1000 deductible, and managed care continues to clip the wings of all types of health care providers.

This rising debt is likely to produce some not so subtle pressures on new graduates that could have far-reaching implications on the integrity and direction of the profession. Besides the bondage that any type of debt has on the borrower, it may blind the least-grounded graduates to make short-sighted decisions. Some will be tempted to sell out to medical interests, beg for table scraps with managed care organizations, or look for acceptance at any cost. If they wanted to be accepted, why did they choose chiropractic?

Patients who still don't understand chiropractic. Perhaps the most profound development of the last decade is that most chiropractic patients are painfully ignorant about chiropractic. Chiropractic was something that merely happened to them, like getting their hair cut. Apparently, during the easy days of insurance, investing in patient education seemed like a waste of time with a seemingly unending supply of new patients waiting in the wings. The sad result are offices facing storage problems from the file folders of patients who enjoyed a brief, low-cost brush with chiropractic, yet found no reason to stay for the maintenance care that most chiropractors, their families, and staff members enjoy on a regular basis.

During this period, many chiropractors abandoned the lectures, educational programs, and family-based practices that had helped chiropractic survive. Instead of producing committed patients who would bail their chiropractor out of jail, the result was a mutant strain of patient, unable to explain chiropractic, defend their decision, or replicate themselves by referring others. The "trophy case" of inactive patients in these offices is a tragic tribute to the myopic, 30-day vision that still guides the decisions of all too many in the profession.

Even in light of the missed opportunities and the 20/20 vision afforded by hindsight, I remain optimistic about the future of the profession. And here's why.

1. This is a profession of fighters. Chiropractic is a profession of independent thinkers who, for the most part, prefer to go against the grain of conventional thinking. The widely-divergent philosophical and practice styles are a curse and a blessing. Yes, they often result in petty infighting, but they reveal a resilient character that will likely help chiropractic survive the challenges ahead.

2. More and more people want chiropractic. A recent study shows that more and more people are fed up with the medical approach of symptom treating and are seeking alternative methods. Not only do they seem to be rejecting the knee-jerk ingestion of high-powered pharmaceuticals, they often get second and third opinions when it comes to surgical interventions. Today, more than ever, chiropractic must remain a distinct healing identity, and not be tempted to become a low-tech modality for the relief of low back pain and headaches.

3. The character assassinations aren't working. The medical boycott has largely gone underground since the Wilk trial and it is considerably less effective. More and more patients are seeing through the baseless political and economic attacks in the media. In many offices, the most profound affect of the *Wall Street Journal* and *20/20* stories was an *increase* in the number of pediatric chiropractic cases! "Oh, I didn't know chiropractors worked with children."

4. The profession is being cleaned up. While no one wants to be the target of professional cleansing, chiropractic, like other professions, has its share of kooks, nut cases, and rip-off artists. These practitioners give chiropractic a black eye and confound the progress of the last decade. The current and future "shake out period" will cause those to leave who got involved in chiropractic for the wrong reasons. This fringe element will migrate to the video rental industry, aluminum siding field, or to multi-level marketing of the latest fad. Good riddance!

5. Chiropractic still works. Even though the last ten years has produced some temporary aberrations, intriguing personalities, fringe elements, and our share of scalawags, chiropractic works as well today than it did 100 years ago. In places around the world where third parties have little or no influence, chiropractic is thriving. Doctors who are infatuated with serving their patients are finding their practices booming. Chiropractors who value chiropractic and are able to communicate its value to patients with passion and creativity, are finding no shortage of new patients. Chiropractic will survive. The only question is, will you be part of it? ■

ADDITIONAL RESOURCES

Again, I was doing a lot of reading during the year this book was written! Here is a list of some of the titles that you might find interesting.

Customer Loyalty, by Jill Griffin. The author offers wonderful insight into the progression and growth of a first time buyer into a loyal, long-term customer. Her continuum starts with "suspects" and "prospects" and culminates in "clients" and "advocates." An excellent book with very clear chiropractic practice implications.

Empires of the Mind, Lessons to Lead and Succeed in a Knowledge-Based World, by Denis Waitley. I enjoy all of Denis Waitley's books and audio cassettes. His gentle spirit revealed here tackles the individual responsibilities we must assume as the Information Age permeates our culture. The notion of leadership as service to those you're leading struck a responsive chord in me. Mr. Waitley explains the often undiscussed and intangible dimensions of patient leadership that I've seen demonstrated in the tableside manners of the most effective chiropractors.

God Wants You To Be Rich, by Paul Zane Pilzer. Okay, the title is a little pandering, but don't let it fool you. Chiropractors unsure of the future would do well to absorb Mr. Pilzer's clearly stated philosophy of abundance. If you're living beyond your means or you need some additional discipline to organize your personal finances, here it is. Regain your optimism for the future!

How To Drive Your Competition Crazy, by Guy Kawasaki. This is one of my favorites on this list. He's made me think more strategically and will probably sharpen your focus, too. Before reading this book our positioning statement at Back Talk Systems, Inc. was simply, "Premier Patient Education." After reading this one we changed it to: "Premier Patient Education For Compliance and Retention." Customer (patient) benefit is everything.

Jesus CEO, Using Ancient Wisdom for Visionary Leadership, by Laurie Beth Jones. The author has explored the gospels and identified almost 100 aspects of effective leadership demonstrated by Jesus. Regardless of your faith, you'll enhance your patient leadership skills by incorporating the simple, but powerful truths in this one!

Jump Start Your Brain, by Doug Hall. If you feel trapped and unable to see the forest for the trees, get a hold of this book. Mr. Hall explains many techniques that can be used to induce creative solutions to just about any challenge or situation. You'll enjoy the real life examples brought from the advertising industry. Fun book.

Living Without A Goal, by James Ogilvy. Certainly the most metaphysical and introspective book on the list, I was first attracted by the title. The author addresses issues that I've seen rarely discussed that deal with our perception of the world and our ability to influence others.

Passion Profit & Power, by Marshall Sylver. This is one of those breezy self-help books, this time written by a professional magician. I found his bold, in-your-face style a little uncomfortable. His incredible energy and passion comes through in each chapter. If you need a serious kick in the pants, grab a highlighter and start rewriting your future.

The 13 Secrets of Power Performance, by Roger Dawson. If you want to change the results (patients, income, staff, etc.) you're getting, the only thing you can really change is yourself. This is a motivational book that explores specific ways you can improve your personal performance, and in turn influence those around you.

The Discipline of Market Leaders, by Michael Treacy and Fred Wiersema. Are you the leading chiropractor in your community? If you're not, you'll find this book interesting. If you are, you'll find this book essential in maintaining and expanding your leadership position. Learn how small mom and pop shops successfully compete when the new Walmart comes to town. (Hint: carve out a niche, instead of trying to be all things to all people!)

The New Positioning, by Jack Trout. This is the follow-up book by one of the guys who helped 7-Up excel by positioning itself as the "uncola" so many years ago. His latest book is full of case histories that you're sure to recognize. Read this book and you'll see why it is critical that chiropractic remain a distinct, healing art, and avoid the temptation to become intoxicated by the medical industrial complex!

The Seven Spiritual Laws of Success, by Deepak Chopra. This little book offers a lot of wisdom that will take a lifetime to appreciate and implement. You can probably read it in one sitting, and then spend years acting on its lessons!

The Wizard of Is, by Tom Thiss. Although not as "new age" as the *Celestine Prophecy*, this book uses an interesting writing style that includes frequently consulting a wise guru that guides the development of the main character. It's a book about self-responsibility and the possibilities that come with it.

The Wow Factory, Creating a Customer Focus Revolution in Your Business, by Paul Levesque. Here's a practical little book about creating extraordinary customer (patient) service. What business are you really in? Find out how to inspire your staff to consistently and systematically exceed patient expectations, the key to positive word-of-mouth advertising.

Turning Lost Customers Into Gold, by Joan Koob Cannie. If you have a trophy case of inactive patients, get this book! How many patients do you lose each year? Why do they drop out? What's the lifetime value of a loyal patient? Have you ever asked your patients what it would take to get them to adopt some type of well-ness/preventive visit schedule?

I mentioned the internet chiro-list newsgroup several times. Subscribing is easy. You'll need a computer, a modem, and access to the internet through either a local provider or a commercial account such as America On Line. Here's what you do: send an e-mail message that reads "subscribe chiro-list" to majordomo@sil-com.com and do not type the quotation marks, change capitalization, add spaces, include your name, or add any other statement or punctuation. (America On Line users need to type chiro-list in the Subject field.) E-mail me at wdesteb@aol.com

William D. Esteb, co-founder of Back Talk Systems, Inc., provides a variety of seminars and communication tools to enhance patient education. Call or write to receive a newsletter and catalog of practice aids that reflect the patient-centered philosophy presented in this book. Mr. Esteb is available for speaking engagements on the topics presented in this and his other books.

For more information contact:

William D. Esteb
Back Talk Systems, Inc.
2845 Ore Mill Drive, Suite 4
Colorado Springs, CO 80904-3161
(719) 633-1165 FAX
(719) 633-1105
(800) 696-1165 FAX
(800) 937-3113